The Miracle Belly Button

Gate to the body – gate to healing

Doris Gföllner

Published by Doris Gföllner, 2022

To my valued readers

When we open the first page of The Miracle Belly Button, we are at the beginning of an extraordinary journey into the world of traditional healing arts. This book is an invitation for you to delve deeper into the ancient wisdom rooted in the practice of Nabhi Chikitsa - a method that nourishes not only the body, but also the mind and soul.

I am deeply honored and inspired by your willingness to embark on this journey. Through this book, it is my sincere desire to shed light on the often overlooked, yet immensely powerful role of the navel in our physical and energetic well-being.

Sharing this ancient practice in modern times, adapted to the needs and challenges of our modern world, has been a journey of discovery and learning for me - a journey that would not have been possible without your openness and interest.

I invite you to contact me with your thoughts, experiences, and insights gained during and after reading this book. Every question, feedback and personal story enriches our shared understanding and appreciation of the healing power that exists within and around us.

If you feel that The Belly Button Miracle has given you new perspectives or useful practices, I welcome any review you would like to leave on Amazon. Your support will help others find their way to this valuable healing practice.

With deep gratitude and in a spirit of connection,

Your Doris Gföllner

Contents

Foreword

Healing via the belly button – it sounds ingenious, and above all it is very simple to practice.

However, it must be borne in mind that not everything can always be "cured" with it. This book does not replace professional advice from a physician or the like. You can wonderfully treat many (almost all) things with it, but often only the symptoms. Oils, for example, which have an anti-inflammatory effect, only help to a limited extent if the cause of the inflammation is not eliminated. One small example: Inflamed rheumatic complaints can of course be greatly improved with various oils, but if you do not change your lifestyle and eating habits, the complaints will not disappear in the long term.

So let this book be an incentive for you to improve your life in all areas. Reduce stress as much as possible, eat a healthy and balanced diet, be thankful for everything in your life Meditate, enjoy the little things in life, your family, your friends, nature...LIFE.

Manifest your life by being HEALTHY and HAPPY. We are very often trapped in what we know. Deeply held beliefs stand in the way of healing. Become aware of your beliefs, change them –

GET READY FOR A HEALTHY BODY AND A WONDERFUL LIFE!

Nabhi Chikitsa – healing through the belly button

It only takes 3 drops of oil in a magical place to improve your health and beauty…

> …and that magical place is your **belly button!!!**

Nabhi Chikitsa means belly button therapy. This traditional healing method is based on the assumption that the belly button takes in and absorbs the essential oil to balance and heal the nerve connections within us. As in all areas of alternative medicine, scientific evidence is lacking.

Nabhi Chikitsa – healing through the belly button – has nevertheless been used for generations and is said to work wonders.

Humans are only created through the connection between their belly button and their mother's circulatory system. We get everything we need to live, blood and nutrients, through the belly button. The belly button is therefore the first contact we have with our mother, through which we get to know our surroundings, our environment, from day one. In Indian Ayurveda, it is therefore known as the part of the body that represents the origin of life. With birth and the cutting of the umbilical cord, we break this connection and become independent beings.

Thus, it stands to reason that the belly button also plays a decisive role after birth. It is a very powerful body part connected to countless nerve endings. In addition, it transmits every stimulation directly to the brain through the very thin and sensitive skin.

Inspired by this information, belly button healing, known in Far Eastern countries as Nabhi Chikitsa, arose.

A therapy that is still used today, especially in India, to support the elimination of physical complaints.

What you should know about the belly button

According to Ayurveda, our belly button is the strongest point that holds the key to the proper functioning of multiple bodily functions.

More than 72,000 veins are connected to the belly button, more than any other part of the human body. This makes the belly button the center of our body. This also explains why applying oils to the belly button can help us to heal numerous health problems in a short period of time. All of these veins help your body function. They support your vision, your metabolism, your circulation, even your hormones. So, give your belly button the attention it deserves. In the western part of the world, we have underestimated this wonderful tool for far too long, even completely forgotten about it.

No wonder that it is an amazing fact that applying oil to the belly button has incredible health and beauty benefits. When we put oil in the belly button, the vein recognizes oil and transports it to the affected parts of the body. There are no side effects of putting oil in the belly button. So, make it a habit to put oil in your belly button every night.

Clean your belly button regularly with mild soap. It is important that you use completely natural soaps, without the addition of chemical ingredients. To thank you for this, your belly button will keep disease-causing germs away from you in return. Stimulate the nerves in your belly button from time to time with a gentle massage. A little pressure with a finger is enough. The massage does not have to last an hour, a few seconds can make a big difference. Take slow, deep breaths and repeat a few times.

Put oil in the belly button and see what happens...

In India, the belly button is one of the most important parts of the body, while in these parts it has been shunted aside. It's small and inconspicuous, but in terms of human origins, we should attach greater importance to.

According to Indian Ayurveda, it should be possible to heal diseases from within by massaging oils into the belly button. Is healing through the belly button an alternative? Try putting oil in your belly button daily and see what happens.

Why the belly button of all things?

It might be strange to hear that our belly buttons can actually perform some magic tricks, but it's no joke! Our belly button is representative of the beginning of our life, and this is where we should return if we want to change our physical health for the better. Did you know that your belly button can help you bring back that lost glow on your face and even heal white patches?

Did you know that your belly button can be a trigger to get rid of acne and even chapped lips? This is all possible when we apply the right natural oils or liquids to our belly button. From cold, flu and menstrual complaints to an increase in fertility, our belly button can work its own special magic as long as we follow a few tips.

How does Nabhi Chikitsa work – healing through the belly button?

First of all, we have to decide on an oil. Of course, that depends entirely on what our complaints are. Each oil unfolds its own specific effect in the belly button.

When we have chapped lips, dry mouth or a runny nose, we still sometimes hear from parents and grandparents that we should put oil in our belly buttons. But does it really do anything?

We often think that it's an ancient belief and we really don't care to trust it. Applying oil to our belly buttons is a simple, effective, and ancient Ayurvedic remedy that has been used as an anti-aging recipe and to cure various common health problems for centuries.

For best results, drip your chosen oil into your belly button right before bed, briefly massage it in and let it work overnight. On the next few pages, you will find a small selection of oils that can support you in strengthening and healing.

Which oils work against which complaints?

A distinction is made here between base oils and essential oils. Of course, you can make all the oils yourself, but that requires a lot of effort. In addition to the ingredients, you also need an oil press and a lot of time to produce a base oil. Distilling essential oils yourself is great if you have the time and the necessary equipment. When buying products, it is important to pay attention to organic quality, and they should not contain any additives. The purer a product, the more effective it is for our body.

Essential oils are very concentrated and can irritate the skin. For this reason, they should only be applied diluted with a base oil. Therefore, only use base oils for children up to school age, as well as during pregnancy. If in doubt, always consult your physician.

If you are unsure about choosing the right oil, you can have it tested or test it yourself. The kinesiological muscle test is ideal for this. Of course, this also works with pendulums and the like, but you have to be open-minded for this type of test. If you already question the test itself, you will inevitably doubt the result. We can block a lot with our thoughts, including successful healing. Therefore, everyone should decide for themselves how to choose the right oil for themselves.

For the essential oils, I have chosen the most important and above all native plants. In my work over the past few decades, treatment with plants from the area where man was born and grew up has proven better than others. For example, many Chinese herbs have a counterpart in Europe. These are the means of MY choice, which is why I'm going to limit this book to them. As you will see below, the right herb for every disease grows here, usually right on our doorstep.

If you use the right belly button oil, the body can benefit from its anti-inflammatory and antioxidant effects.

Correct application

There are 2 types of application:

1. Either you mix a suitable base oil with an essential oil in a ratio of 5:1 or
2. Use 3-5 drops of base oil pure in the navel and then, when the base oil has been massaged in, add 2 drops of essential oil. This protects you from skin irritation caused by the essential oil.

I always recommend, if possible, the 2nd variant. You are more flexible in the combination and you don't have to dispose of any oil mixtures because you haven't used them up. Good oils are not cheap, so you should handle them with care. And essential oils last a very long time, although the base oils can go bad faster.

You can find a recommendation for good essential oils on page 170.

Please be careful with children!

Children under the age of 6 should generally not be given essential oils. And if so, then only in consultation with the pediatrist

Base oils – overview

I use the term base oil to refer to those oils that are obtained by pressing vegetables/nuts/seeds. This requires an oil press and a lot of time. These oils are best produced cold-pressed. When buying, please ensure good organic quality. You can obtain these in every health food store, sometimes also in well-stocked drugstores.

The most important base oils

Peanut oil	Ghee
Coconut oil	Almond oil
Neem oil	Olive oil
Castor oil	Mustard oil
Sesame oil	

Peanut oil

Overview

With its high proportion of mono and polyunsaturated fatty acids, peanut oil has a positive effect on your heart, supports the immune system and has an anti-inflammatory effect.

Origin and properties

Peanuts naturally have a surprisingly high water content of almost 40 percent. Therefore, after harvesting, they are first subjected to a drying process. This lasts between four and six weeks. After that, the water content of the peanuts is only five to seven percent. The peanuts are still in their shells, though. Their fat content is around 45 percent.
In order to get to the fat, the peanuts must first be shelled. Today, this is done by disk mills or corrugated rollers. The peanuts then have to be cleaned of fiber particles and shell residues on vibrating sieves. Then they can be crushed using special roller mills. Now you have ground peanuts, which are better suited for pressing. To extract the contained oil, this mass is now cold pressed with so-called screw presses. In this form, the peanut oil is natural, valuable, intensely flavored and of good quality.

Effect

It is known for its high vitamin E content. In addition, the vitamins B1, D and K are present. Peanut oil has a positive effect on blood pressure, blood fat levels and cholesterol levels. The oil is also said to have a good effect on the immune system and to help with inflammation.
In a medical context, peanut oil can alleviate skin problems. The reason for this is the anti-inflammatory ingredients, but the skin is also

moisturized when nourished with peanut oil. This oil can be used to regulate the metabolism. The omega-3 fatty acids in peanut oil are even said to be able to prevent cancer or alleviate depression.

Peanut oil can bind damaged cell structures in the skin and provide them with moisture. It absorbs well and visibly improves the complexion.
Due to the high content of fatty acids, peanut oil brings cholesterol levels and blood pressure into balance and keeps them in balance.
The high proportion of oleic acid has a positive effect on the heart and blood vessels.
The favorable composition of fatty acids ensures a reduction in blood cholesterol levels and thus a healthy blood lipid level.

The vitamin E in peanut oil protects the body cells from free radicals and strengthens immune defenses. The vitamin E content in peanut oil is high: 100 grams of oil contain around 23.4 milligrams of vitamin E.

Due to the vitamin B1, peanut oil has an effect on the smooth functioning of the thyroid gland.
People who are allergic to peanuts should avoid peanut oil. Allergic reactions can occur as there may be protein residues in the oil. If there is an allergy to peanuts, peanut oil should not be applied to the skin or used as a bath additive. Hair follicles can also become inflamed.

Areas of application

- Age-related itching
- Bowel problems in general
- Bowel obstruction and accumulation of feces in the intestine
- Depression
- Eczema
- Birth – beforehand

- Cancer prevention

- Neurodermatitis

- Abdominal surgery – beforehand

- Rheumatism pain reliever

- Psoriasis

- Metabolism regulating

- Stone-like stool in the rectum

- Dry and scaly skin and scalp

- Poisoning-related multisystem diseases such as multiple hemical sensitivity

- Constipation

Ghee/clarified butter

Overview

Ghee gives moisture to the skin.

According to Ayurveda, the belly button is connected to other parts of the body, so that the moisture should be distributed throughout your body.

Origin and properties

What is ghee? The clarified butterfat is created when butter made from cow or buffalo milk is heated and the solid components (proteins and carbohydrates) are skimmed off the surface.

Effect

It improves blood flow to the nervous system and enhances immunity.

Keeps skin optimally moisturized and improves the complexion.

Prevents skin from drying out and gives the face a natural glow. Heals chapped lips.

Prevents hair loss and keeps it silky and shiny.

Relieves knee and joint pain.

Hides acne and dark spots.

Cures constipation and improves the digestive system.

- Acne spots
- Blood flow to the nervous system
- Hair loss
- Skin spots
- Immune system strengthening
- Knee and joint pain
- Dry skin/lips
- Dry dull hair
- Constipation

Coconut oil

Overview

Massaging coconut oil into the belly button is an ancient Ayurvedic principle.

On the one hand, it keeps your organs healthy and on the other hand it helps avoid gas. The fatty acids it contains curb appetite and increase fat burning. Good news if you want to lose weight. Both its antibacterial and antiviral properties can boost your immune system and thereby prevent infections. Blemishes too should no longer have a chance with this method.

Origin and properties

Coconut oil is a white to yellowish vegetable fat from the nutritive tissue of the coconut and has a very high proportion of saturated fatty acids. It smells very mildly of coconut. It solidifies when the temperature is too cool but liquefies quickly when it is warm. If it is left out too long in the heat, it quickly starts to smell rancid.

Effect

Helps keep our internal organs strong and prevent the body from bloating. Helps treat common symptoms of cough, cold and flu. Relieves stomach cramps during the menstrual cycle. Provides better eyesight. Helps reduce belly fat.

• Applying coconut oil to the belly button is even believed to improve fertility, as the oil contains a medium amount of testosterone which helps to boost fertility in the body.

- Bloated belly
- Cold
- Fertility
- Flu
- Dry skin
- Cough
- Itching
- Dry scalp
- Female cycle cramps
- Sniffles
- Perspiration
- Eyesight

Almond oil

Overview

Almond oil provides a lot of moisture.
Massaging almond oil into your belly button can give your face a real boost of freshness. The facial skin should feel softer and radiate from within. With this method you can counteract both the first signs of aging and blemishes.

Almond oil is a rich source of vitamin E and proteins. By applying 2-3 drops of this oil on the belly button, skin becomes shiny and radiant.

Origin and properties

Almond oil is obtained from sweet almond kernels by cold pressing. The essential (bitter) almond oil is obtained from the kernels of the bitter almonds. Almond oil contains very mild unsaturated fatty acids and vitamin E, which protects skin against cell damage.

Effect

Makes skin shiny and radiant.
Moisturizes skin, leaving it soft and supple.
Reduces dark circles and wrinkles.
Helps heal dry and chapped lips.

- Anti-aging
- Promotes the formation of healthy bacteria in the gut
- Lowers blood pressure
- Improves blood flow
- Anti-inflammatory
- Wrinkles
- Against brittle hair
- Skin – regeneration of damaged
- Skin – keeps it moisturized
- Skin elasticity
- Against dry skin
- Complexion improvement
- Immune system strengthening
- Neurodermatitis
- Osteoporosis – prevention, bone density is preserved
- Helps metabolism to achieve healthier and good insulin production
- Cell damage prevention

Neem oil

Overview

With the oil obtained from the seeds of the Indian neem tree you can put an end to acne. Inflammation of the skin should heal faster. Neem oil is also said to improve the skin structure.

Neem oil is one of the most famous medicinal plants that can heal many skin and health problems.

Origin and properties

Neem oil is extracted from the seeds of the stone fruit of the Indian neem tree. The oil is greenish yellow to brown and smells strongly of onions, garlic and sulfur. The taste is very bitter. It has been scientifically proven that the active ingredients in the oil can kill bacteria, fungi, viruses and mites in humans and animals. The oil also helps against insect larvae, beneficial insects are not harmed.

Effect

Heals pimples and acne. Reduces itching and skin rashes. Helps cure intestinal worms, thereby improving loss of appetite. Used for the treatment of skin infections and eliminates dark spots. Reduces hair loss.

- Acne
- Antibacterial
- Antiviral
- Loss of appetite
- Intestinal worms
- Dark patches of skin
- Eczema
- Fever
- Against ulcers
- Hair loss
- Skin itchy
- Skin rashes
- skin infections
- Herpes
- Itching
- Head lice and dandruff
- Neurodermatitis
- Pimples
- Fungal infections of the skin
- Rheumatism
- Dental hygiene

Olive oil

Overview

This rich oil is the best choice to beat belly fat. Massaging olive oil in and around your belly button every night is said to solve many skin problems and even heal eczema. Olive oil is also said to enhance fertility.

Origin and properties

Olive oil is obtained from the pulp and pits of olives. The taste is mildly bitter. It possesses anti-inflammatory properties, reduces the risk of thrombosis, improves diabetes and lowers blood pressure.

Effect

Improves fertility of women and men.
Stabilizes hormonal imbalance.
Improves male vigor and sperm count.

- Prevents or improves Alzheimer's

- Lowering blood pressure

- Reduces bad cholesterol

- Diabetes

- Anti-inflammatory

- Fertility

- Improves brain power

- Prevents cardiovascular and neurogenerative diseases

- Hormonal imbalances

- Favors calcium absorption

- Bone health

- Cancer preventive

- Prevents or improves osteoporosis

- In pregnant women, it favors the healthy development of the fetus

- Reduces risk of thrombosis

- Prevents tumor formation

- Slows down cell aging

Castor oil

Overview

Castor oil is said to be a particularly good choice for joint pain.

Origin and properties

Castor oil is a vegetable oil obtained from the seeds of the tropical miracle tree. It is colorless to slightly yellowish, transparent and viscous. It tastes mild but very unpleasant and has a strong laxative effect. In addition, it is flammable.

Effect

Reduces swelling of the intestines
Relieves stomach pain and helps against gas
Improves hair growth
Reduces knee pain
Relieves arthritis, back pain and muscle aches

- Age spots
- Arthritis
- Bloated belly
- Intestinal swelling
- Labor induction as a labor cocktail
- Hair loss
- Hair growth
- For firm skin
- Knee pain
- Promotes the skin's own collagen
- Dry lips
- Stomach pain
- Muscle aches
- For healthy nails
- Pigment spots
- Back pain
- Constipation
- Warts (directly on the wart 2x daily)
- For long eyelashes and eyebrows

Mustard oil

Mustard oil is said to be particularly good for cleaning the belly button from dead skin cells and germs. Pain caused by stomach acid or digestive disorders should be combated with mustard oil. If you have puffy eyes or dark circles under your eyes, this oil should be the remedy of choice.

By the way: Mustard oil is extremely moisturizing. It helps, for example, dry and chapped lips to heal, making them soft and wrinkle-free. Simply dabbing a few drops of mustard oil onto your lips can help prevent dry lips in the future.

• Dryness of the skin, especially during the winter season, can be alleviated by applying mustard oil in the belly button.

• If you have long hair, put 3 drops of mustard oil in your belly button every day before you go to sleep.

• Adding mustard oil to your belly button is great for strong and shiny nails.

Origin and properties

Mustard oil is extracted from the mustard seeds of black, white, or brown Indian mustard. It consists largely of monounsaturated fatty acids. When it comes to mustard oil, a distinction must be made between the vegetable oil and the essential oil. We only use vegetable oil here. The oil has a sharp, nutty taste and irritates the sinuses when inhaled due to its sharpness.

Effect

Helps against dry skin, especially due to cold
Keeps lips beautiful and soft, brightens lips with regular use
Strengthens hair and nails
Relieves symptoms of cough, flu, cold and stuffy nose
Improves memory
Reduces fatigue and signs of depression
Heals throat infections and earache
Helps against pain in the legs
Stimulates the bowels and stimulates digestion
Strengthens the immune system and works against bacteria, viruses and fungi
Promotes blood circulation and warms the skin
Relieves muscle tension
Has an analgesic effect
Clears the nose and allows you to breathe more easily
Frees the bronchi of mucus
Stimulates the appetite
Promotes digestion of greasy food
Stimulates the bladder
Relieves rheumatic complaints

Has an anti-inflammatory effect

Gingivitis

Cystitis

Kills fungi and bacteria

Has a disinfecting effect on e.g. cystitis

Risk reduction in cancer

Has an effect against depressive moods

Calming and analgesic effect
on menstrual symptoms

Reduction of headaches associated with menstrual bleeding

- Leg pain
- Cystitis
- Depression
- Cold
- Memory – improved
- Flu
- Sore throats
- Dry skin
- Cough
- Lips brightening
- Lips chapped and dry
- Fatigue
- Muscle tension
- Nails and hair – brittle
- Stuffy nose
- Earache
- Rheumatic complaints
- Expectorant
- Sniffles
- Digestion
- Gingivitis

Sesame oil

Overview

You can use sesame oil to relieve pain and reduce inflammation in joints.

Origin and properties

Sesame oil is extracted from the seeds of the sesame (Sesamum indicum). The light oil obtained from the natural seeds is pale yellow and largely odorless and tasteless – it is mainly used in Asian and Oriental cuisine as an edible oil. It is also used to make margarine [10]. It is a component of skin care products [11] and plays an important role in Ayurveda, where it is used, for example, for forehead oil casting. For the dark sesame oil, the cleaned, hydrated and dried seeds are roasted, pressed after cooling, filtered and bottled. The roasting gives the oil a dark amber color and a typical, intense smell and taste of roasted nuts. This dark sesame oil is not used directly for cooking but is added to dishes in small amounts as a flavoring, especially in Asian cuisine. The production of light sesame oil corresponds to the production of other vegetable oils. Around 300 liters of oil can be obtained from one ton of sesame seeds.

Sesame oil contains valuable antioxidants that strengthen the immune system.

The oil scores with vitamins A and E as well as lecithin. Vitamin A promotes vision and protects the mucous membranes, while vitamin E defuses free radicals, among other things. Lecithin, on the other hand, is important for the function of the brain and nerve cells.

The oil is also characterized by its high proportion of unsaturated fatty acids: It can provide 87 percent unsaturated fatty acids and is therefore very healthy. These fatty acids have a beneficial effect on the cardiovascular system and increase the good HDL cholesterol , while the negative LDL cholesterol decreases.

Linoleic acid in particular is contained in a high proportion: a full 44 percent! Linoleic acid is one of the omega-6 fatty acids. It has a positive effect on heart activity, blood clotting and cholesterol levels. Also, linoleic acid can reduce the risk of arteriosclerosis and osteoporosis.

Areas of application

- Lowers blood lipid levels
- Detoxification
- Purification
- Inflammation
- Prevents osteoporosis and hardening of the arteries
- Teeth – strengthens the structure

As with countless natural healing methods, there is no scientific evidence for Nabhi Chikitsa – healing through the belly button. The lack of research is due to the fact that the often very cost-intensive studies are mainly commissioned by the pharmaceutical companies. Naturally, they have little interest in scientific studies on naturopathic treatments.

Nabhi Chikitsa – healing through the belly button – is a traditional healing method. Passed on through traditions, it is still practiced successfully today – mainly in India. I believe we shouldn't miss the opportunity to become healthy and stay healthy in a natural way.

Essential oils – overview

What is an essential oil?

An essential oil is a mixture of different biochemical compounds that are produced by different plants through their metabolism. These oils are then stored in different parts of the plant in what are known as oil glands.

These essential oils are obtained from herbs, fruits, seeds, twigs, roots, branches, bark, blossoms, leaves, needles or the roots of trees.

Essential oils are liquid substances that are very volatile. This means that they evaporate in air.
If the essential oil is a resinous substance, it is also called resinoid.

Incidentally, essential oils should not be confused with the fatty oil of plants. These fatty oils are, for example, sunflower oil, olive oil, rapeseed oil or linseed oil.

Essential oils are

- mixable with other oils or fats (cream, milk, wax)
- very effective on a physical and psychological level
- very rich in various ingredients
- very intensely scented substances
- not water soluble
- alcohol soluble

The active ingredients have such a small molecular structure that they can penetrate through the skin into the body.

Caution!

Internal use of essential oils can cause serious health problems.

Before using essential oils internally, consult your doctor!

Applying essential oils to the skin can lead to skin irritation!

Only apply diluted essential oils to your skin!

The main essential oils

(native to Europe)

Angelica root	Lavender
Anise	Lemon balm
Arnica	Oregano
Valerian	Peppermint
Basil	Rose
Cistus oil – lemongrass	Rosemary
Dill	Tea tree oil
Fennel	Thyme
St. John's wort	Vanilla
Chamomile	Cinnamon
Pine needle	Lemon

Angelica root

Characteristics

In the Middle Ages, angelica root (angelica archangelica) was a highly valued medicinal plant that, according to Paracelsus, was even used successfully against the plague. Up to 2 m high, the white-flowered umbellifer loves damp, cool locations and is now at home all over Europe. Only plant roots are used for the production of essential angelica root oil.

Effect on the soul

Has a positive effect on anxious, reserved and discouraged people.
Constructive, stabilizing and calming.
Balancing, calming and strengthening for nervousness, sleep disorders and despair.
Dispels negative thoughts, especially after traumatic experiences.

Physical effect

Gas reducing, positive for the heart, antispasmodic, detoxifying, overall physical strengthening, antibacterial, stimulating the immune system, draining, anti-inflammatory, antiviral, circulation strengthening.
Antispasmodic and pain-relieving for stomach disorders, muscle and joint problems. Expectorant and diaphoretic for flu-like infections.
Has a blood-purifying and cardiotonic effect. Bactericidal and fungicidal, strengthens the body's defenses

Balancing, constructive, very calming, gives confidence, gives inner strength, psychologically strengthening, grounding.

- Angina
- Anxiety
- Antibacterial
- Antiseptic
- Arteriosclerosis
- Expectorant
- Gas
- Nervous gas
- Anemia
- Circulatory disorders
- Dyspepsia
- Difficulty falling asleep
- Debloating
- Relaxing
- Vomit
- Exhaustion
- Spring fatigue
- Gastritis
- Flu infection
- Nervous upset stomach
- Stomach pressure
- Stomach ulcers
- Stomach weakness
- Muscle cramps
- Despair
- Nerve strengthening
- Nervousness
- Test anxiety
- Mental and physical weakness
- Motion sickness
- Convalescence
- Rheumatism
- Rheumatism as a rub
- Insomnia
- Sleep disorders
- Expectorant
- Sniffles
- Physical state of weakness

- Flu
- Dermatitis as a compress
- Skin inflammation
- Myocardial insufficiency
- Cardiac insufficiency
- Immune boosting
- Infectious diseases
- Invigorating
- Strengthening
- Paralysis
- Upset stomach
- Sinusitis
- Strengthening after illness
- Stress complaints
- Nausea
- Travel nausea
- Nervous restlessness
- Digestion
- Indigestion
- Dislocations
- Sprains
- Bloating

Anise

Characteristics

Anise has been used as a medicinal plant for centuries because of its excellent antibacterial, expectorant and diuretic properties. A tea infusion made from the seeds of the plant has a particularly soothing effect on complaints of the gastrointestinal tract and respiratory diseases and is also popular with children because of its unobtrusive, slightly sweet taste.

The steam distillation of the seeds produces essential aniseed oil, which is used to treat chronic bronchitis, , sneezing fits, intestinal cramps and gas.

Effect on the soul

Relaxing for nervousness, tension and irritability.
Helps against nightmares and restless sleep.

Physical effect

Has a calming effect, relieves cramps, relieves pain, stimulates the body's fluid production: "Anise lets everything flow," e.g. breast milk, gastric juices or bile juices.
Anise oil has an estrogen-like effect, i.e. balancing and regulating the female hormone balance.
Promotes digestion, antispasmodic and relieving for gastrointestinal

diseases and menstrual cramps.

Expectorant for bronchitis and asthma.

Anti-inflammatory and analgesic for angina.

Diuretic and cardiotonic.

Promotes milk production

slightly antiseptic, antispasmodic, digestive, cardiotonic, expectorant

Psychic or mental effect

Aniseed oil is very calming (sometimes makes you drowsy). It triggers childhood memories of happy days in some people – like folk festivals, Christmas, good candy associated with anise. Relaxing for nervousness. Helps with nightmares. Has a stimulating effect on the mind.

Areas of application

- Asthma
- Difficulty breathing
- Burping
- Gas
- Gas-relieving
- Bronchitis
- Intestinal colic
- Constipation
- Diuretic

- Cough
- Whooping cough
- Colic
- Antispasmodic
- Abdominal pain
- Lung diseases
- Upset stomach
- Menstrual stimulant
- Migraine

- Vomit
- Feet swollen
- Hands swollen
- Nervous heart trouble

- Promotes milk production
- Expectorant
- Metabolism stimulating
- Mucus respiration
- Constipation

Caution

Anise oil contains a lot of trans-anethole. This trans-anethole has an estrogen-like effect and should therefore not be used during pregnancy. However, it can be used after birth to stimulate milk flow.

Under no circumstances is aniseed oil suitable for long-term internal and external use!

Anise oil must be used very sparingly and deliberately, because too high a dosage can cause a numbing, intoxicating effect.

Pregnant women and children are not allowed to use the oil internally!

The oil can irritate the stomach in high doses and cause drowsiness. For this reason, stick to the specified dosage exactly.

Arnica

Characteristics

Arnica oil is one of the best-known medicinal oils. It is used, for example, for ointments, tinctures, in compresses, creams, especially for pain from bruises, sprains or to reduce bruising and limit inflammation or even prevent it altogether.

Arnica oil is rich in silicic acid, which activates and can support our body's self-healing.

Arnica oil furthermore relieves pain in rheumatic diseases, it also helps with insect bites and reduces swelling, inhibits inflammation and has an antiseptic effect.

Arnica oil may only be used externally, and not as a gargle solution if you have inflammation or open wounds in the mouth.

Arnica oil contains ingredients that are toxic and can cause health problems, such as shortness of breath and heart trouble or, in the worst case, to a circulatory collapse.

Internally, arnica may only be taken homeopathically or in ready-made medicines from the pharmacy, because only then can the risk of poisoning be ruled out.

Although arnica is listed among the essential oils here, it is very rare as such. It is usually sold as an oil extract based on a carrier oil. That means you can apply it directly without base oil. You can also prepare the arnica oil extract yourself with your preferred base oil. You can find more information about purchasing and production in the appendix.

Effect on the soul

In case of shock, emotional pain. Releases emotional blockages.
Should be used during (or preferably before) traumatic experiences,
such as separation, operations, exams or a birth.

Physical effect

For bruises and sprains, black and blue marks

Psychic or mental effect

Releases emotional blockages.

Areas of application

- Blood congestion
- Relaxing
- Anti-inflammatory
- Concussion
- Bruises and sprains as an ointment
- Diuretic
- Heart disease
- Liver and spleen swelling
- States of shock

Valerian

Today, valerian oil is mainly used as a general relaxant and sedative. However, valerian also promotes sleep, and it likewise has a calming effect when you are in a state of high excitement.

If you are constantly restless, valerian oil can have a balancing effect. And valerian oil also helps with weather sensitivity, a nervous stomach and other nervous conditions.

In the form of a bath lotion, better as an ingredient, this soothing property can be enjoyed in the most pleasant and relaxing way: Add a few drops of valerian oil to some cream and then add this mixture to the bath water. Have a nice bath.

Valerian oil also alleviates withdrawal symptoms from drug withdrawal, including alcohol withdrawal.

Valerian oil binds gastric acid, so it can also help with stomach pain and heartburn. It has an anti-inflammatory property, especially for eye diseases.

In contrast to other oils, valerian oil does not really play a role in scenting a room because of its peculiar smell, except perhaps in cat rooms.

No other oil has such a calming and relaxing effect on us as valerian oil. It has a soothing effect on us when we are agitated in any way, whether anxiety attacks, stage fright, sleep disorders or constant brooding.

Effect on the soul

Calming, relieves nervousness, relaxes

Physical effect

Valerian inhibits the breakdown of gamma-aminobutyric acid in the brain. When taken in the evening, willingness to sleep is promoted, the time it takes to fall asleep is reduced, the quality of sleep is improved and waking up at night is reduced. When taken during the day, valerian has a calming, relaxing, vegetatively balancing and drive-enhancing effect; it promotes concentration, motivation and the ability to cope with stressful situations and stabilizes the nervous system.

Psychic or mental effect

An interesting aspect is the smell of valerian ("stinkroot"), which is similar to the smell of human perspiration. Current research assumes that the human olfactory brain interprets the scent of valerian as follows: There are other people close to me, so I don't feel alone, but protected and safe.

- Balsamic
- Slightly anesthetic
- Relaxing
- Epilepsy
- Colic and stomach cramps
- Nerve strengthening
- Nervousness
- Sleep inducing
- Insomnia

<u>Basil</u>

Characteristics

Many of us know basil from Italian cuisine. It is one of the most popular herbs that you do not want to be without.

Basil was and still is one of the most important medicinal herbs of Ayurveda, the ancient Indian medicine. Basil probably reached Egypt and Greece via the former Persia, and finally also ancient Rome.

For a long time it was considered a remedy against the so-called "evil eye."

Sometimes basil is also referred to as an aphrodisiac.

Also known in some places as the "royal oil," basil oil strengthens the mind and heart and boosts the body's immune system.

The basil oil is able to improve our memory to improve and sharpen our mind, as was already known to the ancient Indians. Basil oil also helps with nervous disorders, against stress and against fears. It is a natural nerve tonic.

The sweet and herbaceous scent lifts moods during periods of depression and brings clarity to a confused state of mind. It has a stimulating effect on the sympathetic nerves and also strengthens the adrenal cortex.

Basil is also known as a menstrual stimulant and antispasmodic, so it can help against menstrual pain in the form of a compress or as a bath additive and mitigate cramps. But since it also has a stimulating effect, it can be used in the form of a massage mixture to combat fatigue.

Basil oil has also been shown in scientific studies to be effective against acne because it kills the bacteria that promote acne.

In the 16th century, basil leaves were used for inhalations to treat migraines and improve respiratory infections. Basil is used in Ayurvedic medicine this way too, and it also helps against bronchitis, cough and colds, and it is also used as an antidote to poisonous bites. Hindus place sprigs of basil on the chest of the dead to protect them from evil spirits while facilitating the transition between life and death. Women in Italy used to carry the herb with them to win over their loved ones.

Also traditionally used for: Fear, nausea, muscle aches, flu, fever, infections of the lungs and for infectious diseases, as an antidepressant, it is antiseptic and antispasmodic, a digestive tonic and an expectorant. The name basil comes from the Greek basileos = king, meaning it is the kingly herb.

Effect on the soul

Relaxant and tonic for nerves, brain and mind
Balm for mind and soul
Nervous exhaustion
Insomnia
Fear
Sadness

Has a calming and balancing effect, stabilizing, constructive, strengthening, helps against depressive moods, increases concentration.

Physical effect

Very calming, relieves cramps, promotes digestion, dissolves congestion, relieves pain, antifungal, drives away insects.
Mobilizes the sense of smell after sniffles
Expectorant for respiratory diseases
Anti-nausea and antispasmodic for nausea, Gastrointestinal flu and coughing spasms
Virucidal and anti-inflammatory for infections, acne and other skin conditions
Relaxing and analgesic for stress-related headaches
Strengthens the immune system

Psychic or mental effect

Mood-enhancing for anxiety, depressive moods and sadness
Calming and relaxing for insomnia and inner restlessness
Strengthens and invigorates body and mind during stress, exhaustion and nervousness

Areas of application

- Anxiety
- Stimulating on the adrenal cortex
- Antiseptic
- Aphrodisiac

- Stomach problems caused by nerves
- Stomach-strengthening
- Melancholy
- Meno-promoting

- Loss of appetite
- Bronchitis
- Colon cleansing
- Depressive moods
- Relaxing
- Vomit
- Fever
- Mental exhaustion
- Cough
- Insect bites
- Whooping cough
- Headaches and migraines
- Antispasmodic
- Stomach and menstrual cramps
- Nervousness
- Kidney stimulating
- Period too light or absent
- Premenstrual complaints
- Insomnia
- Expectorant
- Sniffles
- Stress
- Toning
- Nausea
- Indigestion
- Warming
- Wash or compress for badly healing wounds

Cistus

Characteristics

Cistus oil has an antiseptic effect, it is astringent and stabilizing. You can use this oil wonderfully for the care of oily skin, e.g. also for acne, or if the skin is inflamed. Cistus oil is said to have been used in creams and ointments as early as ancient Egypt.

Effect on the soul

Cistus oil is invigorating and at the same time soothing, supports meditation and lifts the mood.

Physical effect

It supports the respiratory system, helps to treat wounds, stops bleeding, regenerates the tissue.

Helps a lot against viruses, against bacteria, for cuts in the skin, stops bleeding, relieves coughing irritation, loosens mucus, has a stimulating effect on the lymph nodes, tightens the skin and tissue, regenerates the skin, is highly skin nurturing, positively regulates the vegetative nervous system.

Strengthens the soul and raises it up again, strengthens us internally. Experiences that "went under your skin" are released so that they can be processed.

Relieves emotional coldness.

Areas of application

- Astringent
- Acne
- Acne cosmetic ointments
- Antibacterial
- Antifungal
- Antiseptic
- Antiviral
- Cystitis
- Cystitis baths
- Hemostatic
- Bleeding
- Chronic skin diseases
- Purulent badly healing wounds
- Eczema
- Relaxing
- Decongesting
- Oily skin
- Congested skin
- Mature skin
- Skin diseases
- Skin cancer
- Immunostimulating
- Lymphatic drainage
- Lymph gland swelling
- Lymphatic drainage
- Menstrual stimulant
- Menstrual cramps
- Neurodermatitis
- Psoriasis
- Rubella
- Scarlet fever
- Psoriasis

- Diuretic
- Anti-inflammatory
- Frigidity
- Vessel wall stabilizing
- Tissue regenerating
- Skin inflamed
- Stabilizing
- Stress symptoms
- Toning
- Inner restlessness
- Chickenpox and whooping cough
- Wound healing

Dill

Characteristics

Dill has long been known as a medicinal plant. A tea made from dill is very useful in the treatment of diseases, for example, insomnia.

Effect on the soul

Relaxes, strengthens the spirit and calms the nerves.

Physical effect

The herb is particularly helpful for digestive problems. Many use it to relieve cramps in the uterus, stomach or gut.

Dill has a calming effect on your body, so you can also use the medicinal herb for sleep disorders that may occur.

Dill is also popular during breastfeeding after pregnancy, it stimulates the milk flow in mothers and relieves heartburn.

Psychic or mental effect

Dill is rich in tyrosine, which stimulates the production of dopamine, which in turn floods us with feelings of happiness. It also helps against insomnia and has a stimulating effect on loss of appetite.

- Antiseptic
- Appetite stimulating
- Stomach pain
- Gas
- Debloating
- Relaxing
- Purifies and diuretic
- Vomit
- Nervous vomiting
- Warming

- Antispasmodic
- Gastric and intestinal diseases
- Promotes milk production
- Hiccup
- Digestion
- Digestive promoting
- Warming
- Worms
- Thick mucus in the bronchi

Fennel – sweet fennel

Characteristics

Sweet fennel essential oil is used in aromatherapy to lighten the mood
of the affected person. It has a calming, balancing and energizing
effect on the human soul. Acute stress can thus be mitigated. The soul
is brought back into balance.
Bitter fennel is not palatable!!

Effect on the soul

Fennel can balance and strengthen the psyche. It builds up and
encourages. Orders feelings, creates clarity.
For feelings of abandonment, lack of self-confidence and nervousness,
mental instability. Encourages emotionally cold people to open up.
Mood-brightening during emotional stress, fear of loss and lack of
self-confidence. Energizing for fatigue and lack of drive. Generally
calming and balancing, organizes feelings and brings the soul into
balance

Physical effect

Anti-inflammatory, calming, has an estrogen-like effect, it brings
hormones into balance. This applies to the typical symptoms caused by
menstrual bleeding as well as to symptoms during menopause. Promotes
milk production and relieves cramps. Relaxing and gas-relieving for

indigestion of all kinds. Relaxing for menstrual problems. Anti-inflammatory for angina, abscesses and eye inflammation, blood purifying, diuretic and detoxifying for overweight and urinary stone formation

Psychic or mental effect

Balancing and strengthening

Areas of application

- Antibacterial
- Appetite stimulating
- Eye discomfort
- Stomach pain
- Gas
- Intestinal parasites
- Purifying
- Purification and detoxification of the body
- Cold
- Obesity
- Gout
- Sore throat
- Urinary stones
- Colic
- Cramps
- Lung
- Stomach-strengthening
- Meno-promoting
- Promotes milk production
- Normalizes the menstrual cycle
- Premenstrual complaints
- Expectorant
- Hiccup
- Eyesight strengthening
- Digestion
- Enlargement and tightening of the breast

- Diuretic
- Oily and impure skin
- Cough
- Hangover

- Constipation
- Worming
-

Fennel oil, whether sweet or bitter, may not be used during pregnancy and in the case of epilepsy.

St. John's Wort

Characteristics

Made from the yellow flowers, leaves and stems, St. John's wort oil is best known for its antidepressant and mood-enhancing effects. Also, studies have shown that this oil has a powerful antiviral and anti-inflammatory effect. Useful for minor burns and inflamed areas such as hemorrhoids, varicose veins or nerve pain, great for bruising too.

Effect on the soul

Calming
Effective for stress
Provides support in difficult situations
Mood-brightening for depression and mental stress
Soothing in case of shock, sudden loss and anxiety
Balancing during stress

Physical effect

Analgesic – numbs pain
Anti-allergenic
Antidepressant
Antiseptic
Antiviral
Antioxidant

Bactericidal

Antifungal (Candida)

Anti-inflammatory – reduces inflammation

Antispasmodic

Astringent

Cell regenerative for the skin

Healing of scars

Cooling – cools hot, inflamed areas

Tranquilizer

Immunostimulating

Wound healing

Anti-inflammatory and cooling for hemorrhoids and wound infections

Pain reliever for bruises and muscle aches

Regenerating for skin diseases

Healing for minor burns, scars and wounds

Antiseptic, virucidal and antioxidant, strengthens the immune system

Psychic or mental effect

Helps with:

Fears

Mental shock

Unsolvable problems

Unforeseen losses

Depression

- Circulatory disorders
- Diarrhea
- Anti-inflammatory
- Gout
- Hemorrhoids
- Urinary tract infection
- Sciatica
- Cramps
- Muscle and nerve pain
- Nerve pain
- Nerve strengthening
- Kidney and biliary disorders
- Bruises
- Rheumatism
- Dysentery
- Insomnia
- Painkiller
- Warming
- Wounds
- Wound healing

Caution

St. John's wort oil increases the skin's sensitivity to the light of the sun.

Chamomile

Characteristics

Due to its anti-inflammatory power, chamomile oil is an all-rounder among essential oils.

Chamomile oil helps us in meditation and hypnosis, the oil helps us to let go, it also helps to discard an overly egotistical attitude to life.

Chamomile oil helps us in meditation and hypnosis, the oil helps us to let go, it also helps to discard an overly egotistical attitude to life.

Effect on the soul

Relieves mental cramps.
Relaxing for stress and insomnia
Balancing and calming for excitement, frustration, anger and emotional pressure
Mood-brightening for depression

Physical effect

Antiseptic, bactericidal, antifungal, antimicrobial

Anti-inflammatory – reduces inflammation

Strengthens wound healing

Cell regenerative for the skin, for example in the healing of scars

Cooling – cools a hot, inflamed area

Strengthens the digestive system

Anti-allergenic

Analgesic – numbs pain

Antispasmodic

Anti-inflammatory for abscesses, wounds, burns and cuts

Regenerating for skin diseases and scars

Antispasmodic for menstrual cramps, diarrhea and stomach ailments

Pain reliever for toothache and teething in babies, kidney diseases, nerve pain, migraine and tension

Digestive tonic, diuretic, urinary stone loosening, antipyretic

Has an antibacterial and fungicidal effect

Psychic or mental effect

Relieves stress symptoms.

Provides support in difficult situations.

Calms and relieves anger and frustration.

- Abscesses
- Acne
- General hair care
- Anemia
- Antiseptic
- Lightener for blond hair
- Excitement
- Rash
- Calming
- Conjunctivitis
- Gas
- Burns and cuts
- Burning eyes
- Depression
- Diarrhea
- Problems falling asleep
- Relaxing
- Anti-inflammatory
- Vomit
- Fever
- Fear
- Gastritis
- Vasoconstrictive
- Whooping cough
- Colic compresses
- Headache
- Antispasmodic
- Stomach and intestinal cramps
- Stomach cramps
- Stomach pain
- Massage for tension
- Menotropic baths
- Menstrual stimulant
- Menstrual pain (cramps)
- Migraine
- Mouthwash
- Nerve pain
- Nervousness
- Kidney inflammation
- Earache
- Earache and sore throat
- Rheumatism
- Vaginal catarrh
- Pain-relieving
- Scabs on the scalp
- Stress

- Jaundice
- Stye
- Urinary stones
- Diuretic
- Skin allergies
- Skin inflammation
- Skin itching
- Skin pain
- Hysteria
- Toning
- Indigestion
- Scarring
- Tension
- Wound healing
- Wound irrigation
- Worms
- Teething in young children
- Toothache

Caution

If you are in a treatment with homeopathic remedies, you should not use chamomile oil at the same time.

If the oil has oxidized, i.e. was left in the open air for a long time, it can cause irritation.

Pine needles

Characteristics

Since pine needle oil is highly antibacterial, it can also provide the body with valuable support in strengthening the immune system and fighting off germs. The pain-relieving properties are due to the active ingredient carene.

Effect on the soul

The scent of pine needles strengthens when exhausted and ensures a clear mind. It gives spiritual strength and helps to recharge empty batteries.

Physical effect

It helps against arthritis and many respiratory problems – bronchitis, colds, flu, coronavirus, sore throat and cough as well as sinusitis and runny nose. It relieves urinary tract infections and cystitis. It is a strong expectorant, counteracting congestion of the alveoli, it has a strong antibacterial effect and can therefore even help with severe lung diseases. A clinical study has shown that pine needle oil is particularly effective against the pathogen bacillus tuberculosis. This is what causes tuberculosis.

Pine needle oil inhibits the growth of fungi, which are often the cause of lung ailments and diseases.

The oil has a strong anti-inflammatory effect and is therefore an ideal remedy in the treatment of gastritis. External inflammations of the skin can also be combated effectively.

Internal inflammations, such as rheumatism, can be treated excellently with it as well.

It also has a strong analgesic effect. The active ingredient carene prevents the release of neurotransmitters in the nerves. If these are missing, no pain signal can be transmitted. In this way, it helps against pain in muscles and joints, nerve pain can also be treated well with it.

It is now also being mentioned as a possible antidote to spike protein transmission from people vaccinated for Covid-19 to the unvaccinated.

Psychic or mental effect

The oil has a good effect on exhaustion, nervous exhaustion and stress-related complaints. It promotes concentration and perseverance and even works against depression. It helps to overcome listlessness and lethargy, especially when unpleasant experiences and memories make it difficult for us to move forward with a new life project.

Areas of application

- Decongestant
- Astringent
- Skin reddening
- Impotence

- Stimulating
- Antiseptic
- Alleviating shortness of breath
- Expectorant
- Balsamic
- Bronchitis
- Disinfectant
- Deodorizing
- Anti-inflammatory
- Vasoconstrictive
- Conducive to recovery
- Gout
- Flu
- Diuretic
- Laryngitis
- Invigorating
- Antispasmodic
- Lung infection
- Lung disease
- Sinusitis
- Clogged sinuses
- Rheumatism
- Expectorant
- Diaphoretic
- Spike protein shedding
- Stimulating
- Tuberculosis

Caution

Never use on small children and infants, as it can lead to paralysis of the tongue and, in severe cases, to respiratory paralysis.

Do not use if you suffer from asthma or whooping cough.

Pine oil has a cortisone-like effect, without the drug's side effects.

Lavender

Lavender oil has a liberating effect on our soul, it gives us clear thoughts and helps us to switch off. Lavender oil has a very balancing effect, it refreshes us when we are constantly tired, it brightens our mood, it helps us with nervousness. It also strengthens and calms us, it relieves pain, it has a diuretic and diaphoretic effect. In addition, it has a detoxifying effect, and it helps us to heal wounds faster. The oil also has a strong antiseptic effect.

Areas of application are all diseases of the respiratory organs, earaches, headaches and migraines, gas, diarrhea, nausea, depressive moods, depression, insomnia, nervousness, palpitations, racing heart, high blood pressure, menstrual cramps, childbirth preparation, childbirth, abscesses, acne, skin inflammation, wounds, insect bites, burns, sunburn, muscle strains, sore muscles, sprains, rheumatism, sciatica.

Lavender oil is a very unusual oil with many different ingredients. Lavender oil is very kind to the skin and is good for preparing for labor pains!

Effect on the soul

The oil helps against anxiety, it relaxes the mind, it has a balancing effect against stress. However, it also has a refreshing and invigorating effect on us.
Lavender oil can both calm and stimulate our nervous system, whichever is more important.

That is, it has a balancing effect.
Mood-brightening for depressive moods and mood swings
Calming for anxiety and inner tension
Balancing for irritability and inner restlessness

Physical effect

The oil is particularly antispasmodic as well as calming. It inhibits
inflammation, it helps cell regeneration, it is very healing, especially
for redness or burns. The oil helps against bacteria, against fungal
diseases and it relieves pain.
The notable ester content and the alcohols ensure that the oil is
particularly well tolerated.
Relaxing for stress
Refreshing for exhaustion
Calming and sleep-inducing for nervousness
Pain relief for migraines, strains, rheumatism, bite wounds and cramps
Anti-inflammatory for psoriasis, dermatitis, abscesses and fistulas

Psychic or mental effect

Relieves fears and soothes.
Calming and stress relieving
Mood-brightening
Strengthens the nerves.
Helps relieve tension.
Insomnia
Irritability
Depressive moods
Imbalance
Anxiety and stress

Areas of application

- Abscesses
- Acne
- Anxiety
- Stimulating
- Antidepressant
- Anti-infective
- Antiseptic
- Asthma
- Respiratory diseases
- Constructive
- Balancing
- Leg ulcers
- Calming and stress relieving
- Cystitis
- Blood pressure lowering
- High blood pressure
- Bronchitis
- Cholagogue
- Rosacea
- Dermatitis
- Diarrhea
- Diuretic
- Cardiotonic
- Choleretic
- Hysteria
- Infections
- Infected anal fistulas
- Insect bites
- Whooping cough
- Headache
- Cramps
- Antispasmodic
- Consequences of paralysis
- Lung diseases
- Migraine
- Muscle strains
- Nerve inflammation and sciatica
- Neurasthenia
- Earache and headache
- Psoriasis
- Regenerative
- Stimulates digestive juices
- Motion sickness
- Irritability

- Simple leg ulcers
- Detoxification of the body
- Anti-inflammatory
- Epilepsy
- Cold
- Fever
- Fistulas
- Athlete's foot
- Bile problems
- Ulcers
- Flu
- All skin diseases
- Skin diseases
- Herpes
- Nervous heart trouble
- Rheumatism
- Rheumatic complaints
- Insomnia
- Pain-relieving
- Stretch marks
- Dizziness
- Animal and snake bites
- Gonorrhea
- Typhus
- Burns
- Reduces scarring.
- Growing pains in children
- Leukorrhea
- Wound treatment
- Wounds

Lemon balm

Lemon balm oil stimulates us, but at the same time it can calm us down. It has a very balancing effect on complaints caused by an inner imbalance. Lemon balm oil wards off harmful external influences, it helps us to better relieve tension and regain our inner balance.

Lemon balm oil can almost be described as a protective oil for stressed people, as it has a particularly good and preventive effect against stress.

But lemon balm oil also has a good effect against gas, it lowers blood pressure, it relieves pain, it strengthens digestion, it strengthens the heart, it strengthens the nerves, it relieves cramps, it kills bacteria.

Effect on the soul

Stabilizing for mood swings and depressive moods
Calming for nervous heart problems
Relaxing and sleep-inducing
Refreshing and mood-brightening

Physical effect

This oil works particularly well against viruses, it inhibits inflammation, it stimulates the flow of bile and also the production of gastric juices.

This oil can also help relieve pain and strengthen the body's immune system.

Relaxing and soothing for gastrointestinal diseases, cramps, headaches and rheumatism
Bactericidal and virucidal for inflammation and herpes
Blood pressure lowering and immune-boosting
Hormonally balancing for menopausal symptoms

Psychic or mental effect

This oil calms an excited pounding heart, but it also helps with anxiety, for example when the regular menstrual period is skipped or is too weak due to shock, sadness or fear.
Nightmares
Balancing
In the case of strong mood swings
Calms the nerves
Insomnia
Mood-balancing
Has a balancing and refreshing effect.

Areas of application

- Nightmares
- Allergies
- Anxiety
- Nervous tension

- Immunostimulating
- Insect bites
- Headache
- Cramps

- Antiallergic
- Antibacterial
- Antiviral
- Asthma
- Balancing
- Balancing and refreshing
- Calming
- Calms the nerves
- Bee stings
- Gas
- Anemia
- High blood pressure
- High blood pressure
- Depression
- Decongesting
- Anti-inflammatory
- Bile and liver stimulant
- Vascular regulating
- Strong mood swings
- Tissue tightening
- Oily skin
- Impure skin
- Skin ulcers

- Antispasmodic
- Strong antispasmodic
- Liver and bile diseases
- Liver-biliary diseases
- Gastrointestinal ailments
- Gastrointestinal ailments caused by stress
- Stomach cramps
- Massage oil for migraines and rheumatism
- Menstrual cramps
- Menstrual disorders – menopause
- Migraine
- Plugged ducts
- Night awakening
- Nerve strengthening
- Nervousness
- Mental tension
- Regenerating
- Insomnia
- Insomnia
- Painkiller
- Shock
- Morning sickness
- Dizziness

- Skin care before radiotherapy

- Herpes

- Cold sores

- Herpes diseases

- Heart trouble

- Nervous heart trouble

- Heart problems without organic cause

- Nervous palpitations

- Mood balancing

- Stress relieving

- Stress symptoms

- Irregular menstrual cycle

- Before menstruation

- Menopause

- Sensitivity to weather

Caution

You should not use it during pregnancy or during homeopathic treatment.

Oregano

Characteristics

Oregano oil is considered a natural and powerful antibiotic. Find out here what it helps against and what you should definitely pay attention to when using it.

Oregano is a very popular spice in Italian cuisine, where typical dishes such as pasta and pizza are refined with the aromatic herbs.

But oregano has also been used as a medicinal herb since ancient times. It helps against a variety of health ailments. As a natural antibiotic, you can use oregano oil internally and externally.

Oregano not only grows in the Mediterranean region but is now cultivated in temperate climates around the world. The precious oil is obtained through a steam process. The ingredients may vary slightly depending on the soil conditions.

You can find these ingredients in oregano oil:

Essential oils such as thymol and carvacrol, P-cymene, a powerful pain reliever, vitamins C, B and K, minerals such as iron, potassium, calcium, magnesium and zinc

Oregano oil acts as a powerful natural antibiotic and can be used to treat a variety of health conditions. The oil has an antibacterial, antiviral and fungicidal effect. That is, it fights bacteria, viruses and fungi. In addition, it stimulates blood circulation, is anti-inflammatory and relieves pain. Because oregano oil is rich in antioxidants, cells are protected from free radicals.

The effect of oregano oil can develop best when the medicinal herb has been freshly processed. Dried oregano, for example as a spice, is less aromatic and also loses some of its healing properties.

Effect on the soul

Calming, balancing, brings mental clarity
Strengthens mental resilience
Revitalizing for mental and physical exhaustion
Stimulating for lack of drive

Physical effect

Expectorant and antitussive for chronic bronchitis, tuberculosis and whooping cough
Antispasmodic for acute and chronic asthma
Pain reliever for muscle and joint rheumatism
Strengthens the immune system
Strongly germicidal for infections

Psychic or mental effect

Oregano centers us and helps organize our thoughts. It enables you to distance yourself from many situations and look at them from a different perspective. In this way we come to many new impressions and views that were often seen too one-dimensionally before.

- Acne
- Antibiotic resistance
- Antibiotic
- Bronchitis
- Soothes chemotherapy
- Intestinal parasites
- Stimulates blood circulation
- Inflammation of the gums
- Anti-inflammatory
- Cold
- Impure skin
- Cold sores
- Coughing irritation
- Prevents cancer cell division
- Lice
- Lung infection
- Stimulates gastric juice production
- Strengthens the gastric mucosa
- Tonsillitis
- Multi-resistant germs
- Reduces side effects of chemotherapy
- Earache
- Fungal diseases
- Expectorant
- Pain-relieving
- Inhibits tumor growth
- Digestive-promoting
- Toothache

Caution

Do not use on children under the age of six and pregnant women! Oregano is a member of the Labiatae family and can trigger allergies. If itching, shortness of breath or skin rashes occur in connection with the application, you should consult a doctor immediately.

The oil has a blood thinning effect. If you are taking certain medications, you should only use oregano oil internally after consulting your doctor.

Oregano oil can inhibit the absorption of iron. Therefore, make sure that you take the oil two hours before or after a meal. In addition, you should not exceed the intake period of six weeks. Under no circumstances should you use oregano oil during pregnancy as it can trigger preterm contractions and induce labor!

Peppermint

Mint oil creates clear thoughts and has a refreshing effect, it helps us to reason more, increases concentration, it promotes memory, it relieves cramps and strengthens the immune system, it is antibacterial, it strengthens digestion, inhibits inflammation, it purifies and relieves pain, it promotes blood circulation, it has a diaphoretic and detoxifying effect.
Peppermint oil improves concentration, is stimulating, increases alertness, helps with herpes, increases concentration, is relaxing for our digestive system, helps with nausea, infections, headaches, arthritis, fungal infections(Candida) and rheumatism. It also helps with sprains and insect bites.

Effect on the soul

Refreshes the soul
Frees your mind
Stimulating when exhausted
Refreshing and stimulating
Clarifies thoughts

Physical effect

Anti-inflammatory for infections, prostate and bladder infections, hepatitis and neuralgia

Decongestant and expectorant for respiratory diseases
Strong antispasmodic and analgesic for indigestion, vomiting
and rheumatism
Circulatory stabilization for shock and imminent fainting
Bactericidal, virucidal and fungicidal

Psychic or mental effect

Refreshing
Lack of concentration
Memory enhancing
Mental exhaustion
Enhances concentration
Stimulating

Areas of application

- Defense-enhancing
- Astringent
- Acne
- Anti-infective
- Antiseptic
- Bactericide
- Gas
- Cystitis
- Diarrhea

- Itching
- Headache
- Very strong antispasmodic
- Diseased respiratory system
- Circulatory tonic
- Hepatic and pancreatic weakness
- Stomach-strengthening
- Meno-promoting
- Sore muscles

- Eczema
- Relaxing
- Anti-inflammatory
- Epithelizing
- Vomit
- Cold
- Cold as an inhalation
- Fungicide
- Bile-liver disease
- Ulcers
- Granulation-promoting
- Flu
- Tired impure skin
- Hepatitis
- Herpes
- Palpitations
- Lumbago
- Insect repellent
- Sciatic pain
- Sinus infection
- Nerve inflammation
- Impending fainting
- Bruises
- Prostate inflammation
- Rheumatic pains
- Pain in the head and neck area
- Pain-relieving
- Painkiller
- Shock
- Dizziness
- Sinusitis
- Stimulating on the digestive system
- Nausea
- Virucide
- Wounds
- Wound healing
- Toothache
- Cell renewal

Caution

Do not use on babies and children under 6 years old.
Do not take during the first three months of pregnancy!
Peppermint is a skin irritant!

Do not use during homeopathic treatment!

Can cause dizziness and drowsiness.

Do not use in the evening as peppermint oil can make it difficult to fall asleep.

No internal use during pregnancy!

Rose

Characteristics

The benefits of aromatic oil have been known for a long time, and it is not without reason that rose oil is one of the most expensive among oils. On the one hand, its precious ingredients and the beguiling scent have a positive effect on well-being and appearance. It is also rightly used in the medical field. On the other hand, the extraction of pure oil takes place in a laborious and cost-intensive process.
The aromatic substances of the rose have a harmonizing effect on the psyche. Rose oil helps with insomnia, and it is said to have an antidepressant effect. Already the wonderful scent, which stimulates our synapses via the sense of smell, creates a euphoric mood. For one thing, essential oils – especially rose oil – have an effect on the limbic system in the brain via their aromatic scent and can have a positive influence on mood there. For another, they are able to penetrate skin layers to develop their effect both in the body and on the skin. That is why the oil is used to the full extent in skin care. Its antiseptic properties have a supporting effect here. Because it promotes wound healing, it is also good for small wounds and inflammation. It counteracts physical complaints in that it relieves pain and tension as well as releases cramps.

Effect on the soul

Calming for nervousness
Stimulating when exhausted

Mood-brightening for depression and disappointments
Stabilizing for mental trauma and shock
Aphrodisiac

Physical effect

Anti-inflammatory for shingles, bronchitis, , gum and eye
inflammation
Pain reliever during childbirth
Nurturing and regenerating for chronic skin diseases, wounds
and irritation
Relaxing for sore muscles, menstrual and digestive problems
Heart strengthening and sleep-inducing

Psychic or mental effect

The delicate scent of rose oil has an extremely positive influence on our
psyche. It is considered a mood enhancer and is widely used to treat
depression and to combat depressive moods. Furthermore, rose oil has a
strong relaxing and balancing effect. This means that, for example, in
the event of inner restlessness, tension and general nervousness, the oil
positively influences and balances our psyche.
For sleep disorders due to inner restlessness and tension, the rose oil has
a balancing effect and helps to achieve a natural sleep. But beware!
Rose oil can help also have a stimulating effect with fatigue due to its
balancing effect. It should therefore primarily balance restlessness and
tension and not be used for general sleep disorders.

- Anxiety and stressful conditions
- Antibacterial
- Antiseptic
- Bronchitis and sore throat
- Depression
- Stimulates blood circulation
- Relaxing for tension
- Anti-inflammatory
- Moisturizing
- Headache
- Antispasmodic
- Menstrual cramps
- Migraine
- Fatigue
- Pain-relieving
- Promotes wound healing
- Gingivitis
- Cell renewal

Rosemary

Characteristics

The essential oils in rosemary have been said to have healing and health-promoting effects since ancient times. Precious rosemary oil can be produced from the sprigs of rosemary, which you can use wonderfully in the kitchen or as a healing oil.

Effect on the soul

Stimulating for apathy and mental exhaustion
Invigorating for weakness
Promotes self-confidence and resilience

Physical effect

Pain reliever for muscle and joint problems and neuralgia
Increases blood pressure for hypotension
Strengthens the cardiovascular system
Promotes digestion, liver activity and bile flow
Expectorant for colds
Stimulates blood circulation during athletic exertion
Strengthens the immune system

Psychic or mental effect

Rosemary promotes mental activity, concentration and brain function. Studies have proven that inhaling rosemary oil makes you more productive.
Counteracts stress and relieves nervous tension. Rosemary oil helps so well against stress because it lowers the stress hormone cortisol, giving the oil a calming effect.

Areas of application

- Antibacterial
- Listlessness
- Gas
- Cholesterol reducing
- Depression
- Diet supportive
- Colds
- Increasing memory performance
- Tachycardia caused by low blood pressure
- Cardiac arrhythmias caused by low blood pressure
- Infections
- Dizziness from low blood pressure
- Mood swings
- Stress
- Nausea
- Restlessness
- Improvement of liver and bile activity
- Constipation
- Wound healing

For epilepsy and pregnancy do not use essential rosemary oil
(promotes menstruation)
Since the essential oil also works against low blood pressure,
you should avoid its use with high blood pressure as well.

Tea tree – manuka

Characteristics

Manuka (leptospermum scoparium) is a plant of the myrtle family and is one of the traditional medicinal plants in New Zealand. Only the manuka tree has the active ingredient leptospermum, which has a much stronger bactericidal and fungicidal effect than tea tree oil but is just as skin-friendly. Manuka essential oil uses leaves and twigs.

Effect on the soul

Relaxing for nervous restlessness and mental exhaustion
Stimulating when exhausted and overwhelmed
Stimulates the mind and clarifies thoughts
Calming for anxiety and nervousness
Alleviates psychosomatic complaints
Strengthening and uplifting in unstable emotional state, stress and overwhelm
Soothing for psychosomatic illnesses
Dampens the excessive release of stress hormones

Physical effect

Strengthens the immune system.
Anti-inflammatory, healing and antipruritic for wounds, dental problems, fungus, neurodermatitis and insect bites.

Anti-inflammatory for eczema, respiratory diseases, acne and urinary tract infections. Antipruritic and soothing for acne, psoriasis, eczema and scar growths. Expectorant for respiratory diseases.
Pain-relieving and blood circulation-promoting for sore muscles. Pain reliever for muscle tension and rheumatism.
Fungicide and virucidal for fungal diseases, warts and herpes
Bactericide for gingivitis and blemishes
Strengthens the immune system

Psychic or mental effect

A high proportion of "skin and soul comforting" alcohols helps with anxiety and strengthens self-confidence.
Supplies strength and determination when the soul is out of balance and brings clarity to feelings and thoughts.
Tea tree oil has a cleansing, clarifying, strengthening and balancing effect and helps with listlessness, lack of drive and states of exhaustion. Tea tree oil helps especially sensitive people who are quickly affected by stress and anxiety in their stomach.

Areas of application

- Antibacterial
- Soothes the scalp
- Inflammation
- Anti-inflammatory
- Cold

- Itching
- Head lice
- Dandruff
- Mites
- Bad breath

- Fleas
- Athlete's foot
- Foot perspiration
- Sore throat
- Skin diseases and blemishes
- Herpes
- Infections
- Insect bites
- Nail fungus
- Fungicidal
- Sniffles
- Warts
- Supports wound healing
- Gingivitis
- Ticks

Thyme

Characteristics

Thyme oil (thymus vulgaris)

Thyme originally comes from the Mediterranean region, but is now grown in our gardens too.

The Greek word "thymus" means something like "courage," and that was probably also the reason why thyme was placed on the heads of soldiers in ancient Greece in the form of a wreath when they went to war.

Thyme came to us from the Mediterranean region in the 11th century, it was the monks who brought it from the south because of its wonderful effects. Thyme was grown in monastery gardens and its healing properties for all sorts of illnesses were discovered fairly quickly. It was Hildegard von Bingen, for example, who was one of the first to write about the healing properties of thyme.

Even today, thyme is used for coughs , for example used, but of course it is also a spice that makes our food tastier and more palatable.

The essential oil of thyme is obtained through steam distillation, it smells very spicy and intense.

Thyme is antimicrobial, cleansing, antiparasitic, antifungal, disinfectant, antiviral. Thyme oil helps with bronchitis, vascular diseases, Alzheimer's, coughs, hepatitis, heart disease, dry cough, infectious diseases.

Thyme oil invigorates, so that it helps with exhaustion or else after a long illness.

Thyme oil gives us strength and courage, it strengthens our self-confidence.

Thyme oil is also antiseptic, it relieves cramps and mucus, it
increases the body's own defenses, it promotes blood circulation,
it increases appetite and is good for digestion. In addition, it has
a blood pressure increasing effect.

Effect on the soul

Strengthening for mental stress
Promotes courage and determination
Calming for anxiety, insomnia and weak nerves

Physical effect

The essential oil of thyme, thymol, has a strong disinfecting effect, it
gives strength and has a constructive and strengthening effect. It
serves as an effective aid and protective shield for a weakened
constitution, emerging infections and colds.
Analgesic and warming for arthritis, neuralgia, circulatory disorders
and rheumatism
Antispasmodic and digestive tonic for gastrointestinal diseases
Expectorant for colds, whooping cough, asthma and tuberculosis

Increases blood pressure, promotes blood circulation
Antiseptic, strengthens the immune system

Strengthens in case of mental weakness.
Supplies courage to act.
Gives warmth and compassion.

Areas of application

- Strengthening the immune system in infectious diseases
- Anxiety
- Antirheumatic
- Antiseptic
- Appetite stimulating
- Arthritis
- Anemia
- Blood pressure increasing
- Bronchitis
- Stimulates blood circulation
- Cold
- Exhaustion
- Cough
- Immune and nerve weakness
- Intelligence stimulating
- Capillary circulation
- Whooping cough
- Antispasmodic
- Circulatory disorder
- Gastrointestinal infection
- Stomach-strengthening
- Meno-promoting
- Nerve pain
- Rheumatism
- Insomnia
- Expectorant
- Weakness
- Strengthening
- Tuberculosis
- Digestion
- Worming

Warning in case of hyperthyroidism and high blood pressure!

Do not use with epilepsy!

During pregnancy or if you have high blood pressure, the oil must not be used.

Do not use thyme essential oil in pregnancy, epilepsy, hyperthyroidism and high blood pressure!

Vanilla

Characteristics

Because vanilla can act so directly on our emotional center, it is not surprising that it is used in aromatherapy against diseases that can upend our emotional worlds: diseases such as depression, anxiety disorders and stress, to name just the most important ones.

Effect on the soul

Soothing and calming.
Reminiscent of Christmas or Advent.
The scent will break any ice.
Gives comfort.
Relaxing for stress
Mood-brightening for depression
Calming for sleep disorders, restlessness and anxiety
Balancing for rage, anger and frustration
Stimulating for lethargy and fatigue
Relaxing for stress
Mood-brightening for depression
Calming for insomnia, restlessness and anxiety
Balancing for rage, anger and frustration
Stimulating for lethargy and fatigue

Physical effect

Pain-relieving and relaxing for sore muscles
Fungicide for fungal diseases
Digestive and menstrual tonic
Antispasmodic for indigestion
Anti-inflammatory for neurodermatitis
Skin conditioning and antioxidant
Pain-relieving and relaxing for sore muscles
Fungicide for fungal diseases
Digestive and menstrual tonic
Antispasmodic for indigestion
Anti-inflammatory for neurodermatitis
Skin conditioning and antioxidant

Psychic or mental effect

Vanilla gives the cuddly feeling of security. Breast milk
smells slightly of vanilla.

Areas of application

- Anxiety
- Stimulating for digestion
- Antiseptic
- Aphrodisiac
- Germicidal
- Slight menstrual tonic
- Neurodermatitis
- Fungal diseases of the skin

- Anger calming
- Diet-accompanying – inhibits the desire for sweets
- Relaxing
- Anti-inflammatory
- Frustration
- Mental tension
- Sexual problems
- Mood-brightening
- Anger

Caution

Warning: Do not use essential vanilla oil during pregnancy, it promotes menstruation!

Cinnamon

Characteristics

When I talk about cinnamon oil, I always mean cinnamon bark oil.

Cinnamon was prized by the ancient Egyptians and has been used by Chinese and Ayurvedic practitioners in Asia for thousands of years to treat everything from depression to weight gain. Whether as a spice, in tea or in herbal form, cinnamon has been helping people for centuries.

Effect on the soul

Promotes motivation, vitality, creativity and a positive attitude towards life
Conveys a feeling of protection and security
Stimulating and aphrodisiac

Physical effect

Many of the benefits of cinnamon bark oil are related to its ability to dilate blood vessels. Cinnamon bark may help improve nitric oxide function, resulting in increased blood flow and reduced inflammation.
Warming for influenza infections
Stimulating when exhausted
Mood-brightening during depressive phases

Pain reliever for rheumatism and sore muscles
Can increase blood pressure, strengthens the immune system and lowers blood sugar levels in diabetes
Strongly bactericidal and virucidal

Psychic or mental effect

Cinnamon is an important remedy for people who are emotionally oversensitive. The strong tonic increases cardiac and pulmonary performance and is therefore excellently suited in the case of weakness after flu infections.

Areas of application

- Antibacterial
- Loss of appetite
- Gas
- Dilates blood vessels
- Hemostatic
- Hemostatic for nosebleeds and heavy menstrual bleeding
- Regulates blood sugar
- Balances cholesterol
- Depression
- Diabetes
- Diarrhea

- Immune boosting
- Infections
- Catarrhal congestion
- Colic
- Stimulates libido
- Nail fungus
- Parasites
- Rheumatism
- Weak digestion
- Heavy menstrual bleeding
- Enhancing metabolism

- Detoxification
- Anti-inflammatory
- Vomit
- Fungicide
- Cardiotonic

- Nausea
- Overweight
- Digestive-promoting
- Constipation

Caution

Do not use during pregnancy and breastfeeding or in children under the age of five! Cinnamon from the cinnamon tree contains coumarin, a chemical that can cause liver and kidney damage and worsen liver disease if too much is used.

Lemon

Characteristics

The lemon became particularly popular in Europe when it became clear that the vitamins contained in it were effective against scurvy, one of the most terrible diseases in the Middle Ages, especially among seafarers. However, the lemon can do even more, as even people back then quickly discovered: It also helps against fever caused by infections, digestive problems, skin problems, arthritis and can be used for skin care.

Lemon oil is very strong cleansing, antibacterial, antitumor, antiseptic. It purifies, has a relaxing effect, it helps with arteriosclerosis, increases the ability to concentrate, it helps with circulatory problems, has an antidepressant effect, brightens moods, enhances memory, helps against warts, strengthens our immune system, it helps with infections of all kinds, it also helps with digestive problems.

Effect on the soul

Gives lightness and freshness
Calming balancing for anxiety and compulsive brooding
Stimulating for fatigue, weakness and stress
Mood-brightening, promotes dopamine release

Physical effect

Hemostatic, anti-inflammatory, antipyretic, diuretic, heart tonic, antispasmodic, promotes concentration, mentally stimulating, mood-brightening, antianemic, antimicrobial, antirheumatic, antisclerotic, antiseptic, antibacterial, digestive tonic, immune-enhancing
Stimulating for bile discharge, antibacterial (especially streptococci), antifungal, antiviral, gas, anti-inflammatory, antipyretic, herpes, respiratory infections, varicose veins, liver weakness, liver tonic, tonsillitis, convalescence, stagnation of bile flow, strong antiseptic (ambient air), metabolism stimulating, thrombosis, venous insufficiency, vein tonic, diaphoretic, diuretic, antipyretic, hemostatic, hypotensive, insecticidal, astringent, antiseptic, brittle nails, purifying, oily skin, broken capillaries, congested skin, freckles

Psychic or mental effect

Stimulating, concentration-enhancing, mood-brightening, stress-relieving, revitalizing

Areas of application

- Signs of aging
- Anemia
- Angina
- Antibacterial
- Arteriosclerosis

- Sore throat
- Hands swollen
- Oily skin
- Oily and impure skin
- Skin rashes

- Arthritis
- Asthma
- Conjunctivitis
- Blood pressure lowering
- Bruising
- High blood pressure
- Blood cleansing
- Hemostatic
- Bowel detox
- Intestinal inflammation
- Intestinal catarrh
- General intestinal diseases
- Demineralization
- Depressive moods
- Colon inflammation
- Inflammation of the small intestine
- Purifying
- Diuretic
- Vomit
- Cold
- Obesity
- Fever
- Scaly patches
- General skin problems
- Hoarseness
- Herpes
- Infections
- Itching
- Difficulty concentrating
- Strengthens the gums as a mouthwash
- Varicose veins
- Liver disease
- Lung diseases
- Stomach ulcers
- Gastric acidity
- Migraine
- Mouth ulcers
- Weeping rashes
- Rheumatism
- Chills
- Physical and mental weaknesses
- Swelling
- Low self-confidence
- Scurvy
- Metabolism boosting
- Metabolic disorders

- Boils
- Feet swollen
- Gallstones
- Broken capillaries
- Gout
- Flu infection
- Flu
- Throat infections
- Acidification of the body
- Vein problems
- Phlebitis
- Venous congestion
- Digestion
- Prevention against colds
- Warts
- Wounds
- Gingivitis

Caution

Lemon oil is a mild skin irritant. For external use, you should always follow the dosage instructions. When exposed to the sun, irritation can occur on skin treated with lemon oil.

Overview effect of base oils according to symptoms

P=peanut oil, G=ghee, Co=coconut oil, A=almond oil, N=neem oil, O=olive oil, Ca=castor oil, M=mustard oil, S=sesame oil								
Abdominal surgery – beforehand	P							
Acne					N			
Acne spots		G						
Against brittle hair				A				
Against dry skin				A				
Against ulcers					N			
Age spots							Ca	
Age-related itching	P							
Anti-aging				A				
Anti-inflammatory				A		O		
Antibacterial and antiviral effect					N			
Arthritis							Ca	
Back pain							Ca	
Bacteria in the gut – promotes the formation of healthy				A				
Birth – beforehand	P							
Bloated belly			Co					
Blood flow to the nervous system		G						
Blood lipid level reduction								S
Bowel problems in general	P							

Condition	P	G	Co	A	N	O	Ca	M	S
Cancer preventive						O			
Cold			Co					M	
Collagen – promotes the skin's own							Ca		
Complexion improvement				A					
Constipation	P	G					Ca		
Cough			Co					M	
Cystitis									S
Dark patches of skin					N				
Depression	P							M	
Detoxification									S
Diabetes						O			
Digestion								M	
Dry and scaly skin and scalp	P								
Dry dull hair		G							
Dry skin/lips		G							
Earache								M	
Eczema	P				N				
Expectorant								M	
Eyesight			Co						
Fatigue								M	
Favors calcium absorption and thus bone health						O			
Female cycle cramps			Co						

P=peanut oil, G=ghee, Co=coconut oil, A=almond oil, N=neem oil, O=olive oil, Ca=castor oil, M=mustard oil, S=sesame oil

P=peanut oil, G=ghee, Co=coconut oil, A=almond oil, N=neem oil, O=olive oil, Ca=castor oil, M=mustard oil, S=sesame oil								
Fertility			Co			O		
Fever					N			
Flu			Co					M
Fungal infections of the skin					N			
Gas							Ca	
Hair growth							Ca	
Hair loss		G			N		Ca	
Head lice and dandruff					N			
Herpes					N			
Hormonal imbalances						O		
Immune system strengthening		G		A				
Improve brain power						O		
Improving blood flow				A				
In pregnant women, favors the healthy development of the fetus						O		
Inflammation									S
Intestinal obstruction and accumulation of feces in the intestine	P							
Intestinal swelling							Ca	
Intestinal worms					N			
Itch relief			Co					
Itching					N			
Knee and joint pain		G						

P=peanut oil, G=ghee, Co=coconut oil, A=almond oil, N=neem oil, O=olive oil, Ca=castor oil, M=mustard oil, S=sesame oil								
knee pain							Ca		
Labor induction as a labor cocktail							Ca		
Leg pain									S
Lips brightening								M	
Lips chapped and dry								M	
Lips dry							Ca		
Loss of appetite					N				
Lowering blood pressure				A		O			
Memory – improved								M	
Metabolism – helps to have a healthier and good insulin production				A					
Metabolism regulating	P								
Muscle aches							Ca		
Muscle tension								M	
Nails and hair – brittle								M	
Nails, healthy							Ca		
Neurodermatitis	P			A	N				
Osteoporosis – prevention, bone density is preserved				A					
Perspiration			Co						
Pigment spots							Ca		
Pimples					N				
Poisoning-related multisystem diseases such as multiple chemical sensitivity	P								

P=peanut oil, G=ghee, Co=coconut oil, A=almond oil, N=neem oil, O=olive oil, Ca=castor oil, M=mustard oil, S=sesame oil								
Prevent or improve Alzheimer's						O		
Prevent or improve osteoporosis						O		
Prevent tumor formation						O		
Prevention against cancer diseases	P							
Prevents cardiovascular and neurogenerative diseases						O		
Prevents osteoporosis and hardening of the arteries									S
Psoriasis	P							
Purification									S
Reduce risk of thrombosis						O		
Reduces bad cholesterol						O		
Rheumatic complaints								M
Rheumatism					N			
Rheumatism pain reliever	P							
Scalp dry			Co					
Skin – keeps it moisturized				A				
Skin – regeneration of damaged				A				
Skin dry			Co					M
Skin elasticity				A				
Skin for firm							Ca	
Skin infections					N			
Skin itchy					N			
Skin rashes					N			

P=peanut oil, G=ghee, Co=coconut oil, A=almond oil, N=neem oil, O=olive oil, Ca=castor oil, M=mustard oil, S=sesame oil									
Skin spots		G							
Sniffles			Co					M	
Sore throats								M	
Stomach pain							Ca		
Stone-like stool in the rectum	P								
Stuffy nose								M	
Warts (directly on the wart 2x daily)							Ca		
Wrinkles				A					

Overview of effects of essential oils according to symptoms

	Abdominal pain	Abscesses	Acne	Acne cosmetic	Adrenal cortex	Allergies	Alleviate side effects of chemotherapy
Angelica root							
Anise	X						
Arnica							
Basil					X		
Chamomile		X	X				
Cinnamon							
Cistus oil – lemongrass			X	X			
Dill							
Fennel							
Lavender		X	X				
Lemon							
Lemon balm			X			X	
Oregano			X				X
Peppermint			X				
Pine needle							
Rose							
Rosemary							
St. John's wort							
Tea tree oil							
Thyme							
Valerian							
Vanilla							

	Anemia	Anesthetic slight	Anger	Anger calming	Angina	Animal and snake bites	Antiallergic	Antibacterial	Antibiotic
Angelica root					X			X	
Anise									
Arnica									
Basil									
Chamomile	X								
Cinnamon								X	
Cistus oil – lemongrass								X	
Dill									
Fennel								X	
Lavender						X			
Lemon	X				X			X	
Lemon balm							X	X	
Oregano									X
Peppermint									
Pine needle									
Rose								X	
Rosemary								X	
St. John's wort									
Tea tree oil								X	
Thyme									
Valerian		X							
Vanilla			X	X					

	Anticonvulsant	Antidepressant	Antifungal	Anti-gas	Antihypertensive	Anti-infectious	Anti-inflammatory	Antirheumatic	Antiseptic	Antispasmodic
Angelica root	X			X					X	
Anise										X
Arnica	X						X			
Basil	X								X	X
Chamomile							X		X	X
Cinnamon							X			
Cistus oil – lemongrass	X		X				X		X	
Dill	X			X					X	
Fennel										
Lavender		X			X	X	X		X	X
Lemon					X					
Lemon balm							X			X
Oregano							X			
Peppermint	X					X	X		X	
Pine needle							X		X	X
Rose							X		X	X
Rosemary										
St. John's wort							X			
Tea tree oil							X			
Thyme								X	X	X
Valerian	X									
Vanilla							X		X	

	Antispasmodic strong	Antiviral	Anxiety	Anxiety and stress	Aphrodisiac	Appetite-promoting	Arthritis	Asthma	Astringent
Angelica root			X						
Anise								X	
Arnica									
Basil			X		X				
Chamomile									
Cinnamon									
Cistus oil – lemongrass		X							X
Dill						X			
Fennel						X			
Lavender			X					X	
Lemon							X	X	
Lemon balm	X	X	X					X	X
Oregano									
Peppermint	X								X
Pine needle									X
Rose					X				
Rosemary									
St. John's wort									
Tea tree oil									
Thyme			X			X	X		
Valerian									
Vanilla			X		X				

	Atherosclerosis	Athlete's foot	Bactericidal	Bad Breath	Balancing	Balancing and refreshing	Balsamic	Barleycorn	Bee stings	Before menstruation
Angelica root	X									
Anise										
Arnica										
Basil										
Chamomile								X		
Cinnamon										
Cistus oil – lemongrass										
Dill										
Fennel										
Lavender		X			X					
Lemon	X									
Lemon balm					X	X			X	X
Oregano										
Peppermint			X							
Pine needle							X			
Rose										
Rosemary										
St. John's wort										
Tea tree oil		X		X						
Thyme										
Valerian							X			
Vanilla										

	Bile and liver stimulant	Bile disorders	Biliary liver disease	Bladder infection	Bleeding	Bloating	Blonde hair lightener	Blood pressure high	Blood pressure increase	Blood purifier
Angelica root						X				
Anise										
Arnica										
Basil										
Chamomile							X			
Cinnamon										
Cistus oil – lemongrass					X					
Dill										
Fennel										
Lavender		X								
Lemon										X
Lemon balm	X							X		
Oregano										
Peppermint			X							
Pine needle										
Rose										
Rosemary										
St. John's wort				X						
Tea tree oil										
Thyme									X	
Valerian										
Vanilla										

	Blood sugar regulating	Blood vessel dilating	Body detox	Boils	Boost gastric juice production	Breast enlargement and firming	Broken veins	Bronchitis	Bronchitis and sore throat
Angelica root									
Anise								X	
Arnica									
Basil								X	
Chamomile									
Cinnamon	X	X							
Cistus oil – lemongrass									
Dill									
Fennel						X			
Lavender			X					X	
Lemon				X			X		
Lemon balm									
Oregano					X			X	
Peppermint									
Pine needle								X	
Rose									X
Rosemary									
St. John's wort									
Tea tree oil									
Thyme								X	
Valerian									
Vanilla									

	Bruises	Bruises and sprains as an ointment	Burning eyes	Burns	Burns and cuts	Burping	Calming and stress relieving	Calms the nerves	Capillary circulation
Angelica root									
Anise						X			
Arnica		X							
Basil									
Chamomile			X		X				
Cinnamon									
Cistus oil – lemongrass									
Dill									
Fennel									
Lavender				X			X		
Lemon	X								
Lemon balm								X	
Oregano									
Peppermint	X								
Pine needle									
Rose									
Rosemary									
St. John's wort	X								
Tea tree oil									
Thyme									X
Valerian									
Vanilla									

	Cardiac arrhythmias caused by low blood pressure	Cardiotonic	Catarrhal congestion	Cell renewal	Chemotherapy relief	Chickenpox and whooping cough	Children's growing pains	Chills
Angelica root								
Anise								
Arnica								
Basil								
Chamomile								
Cinnamon		X	X					
Cistus oil – lemongrass						X		
Dill								
Fennel								
Lavender		X					X	
Lemon								X
Lemon balm								
Oregano					X			
Peppermint				X				
Pine needle								
Rose				X				
Rosemary	X							
St. John's wort								
Tea tree oil								
Thyme								
Valerian								
Vanilla								

	Cholagogue	Choleretic	Cholesterol balancing	Cholesterol reducing	Chronic skin diseases	Circulatory	Circulatory disorders	Cold	Cold as an inhalation	Cold sore
Angelica root							X	X		
Anise										
Arnica										
Basil								X		
Chamomile										
Cinnamon			X							
Cistus oil – lemongrass					X					
Dill										
Fennel								X		
Lavender	X	X						X		
Lemon								X		
Lemon balm										X
Oregano								X		X
Peppermint						X		X	X	
Pine needle										
Rose										
Rosemary				X						
St. John's wort							X			
Tea tree oil								X		
Thyme							X	X		
Valerian										
Vanilla										

	Colds	Colic	Colic compresses	Colic and stomach cramps	Colon cleanse	Colon detox	Colon inflammation	Concussion	Congestion
Angelica root									
Anise		X							
Arnica								X	X
Basil					X				
Chamomile			X						
Cinnamon		X							
Cistus oil – lemongrass									
Dill									
Fennel		X							
Lavender									
Lemon						X	X		
Lemon balm									
Oregano									
Peppermint									
Pine needle									
Rose									
Rosemary	X								
St. John's wort									
Tea tree oil									
Thyme									
Valerian				X					
Vanilla									

	Conjunctivitis	Consequences of paralysis	Constipation	Convalescence	Cough	Cough stimulus	Cramps	Cystitis	Cystitis baths
Angelica root				X					
Anise			X		X				
Arnica									
Basil					X				
Chamomile	X								
Cinnamon			X						
Cistus oil – lemongrass								X	X
Dill									
Fennel			X		X		X		
Lavender		X					X	X	
Lemon	X								
Lemon balm							X		
Oregano						X			
Peppermint								X	
Pine needle									
Rose									
Rosemary			X						
St. John's wort							X		
Tea tree oil									
Thyme					X				
Valerian									
Vanilla									

	Dandruff	Decongestant	Decongesting	Defense-enhancing	Demineralization	Deodorant	Depression	Depressive moods	Dermatitis	Dermatitis as a compress
Angelica root										X
Anise										
Arnica										
Basil								X		
Chamomile							X			
Cinnamon							X			
Cistus oil – lemongrass			X							
Dill										
Fennel										
Lavender									X	
Lemon				X				X		
Lemon balm			X				X			
Oregano										
Peppermint				X						
Pine needle		X				X				
Rose							X			
Rosemary							X			
St. John's wort										
Tea tree oil	X									
Thyme										
Valerian										
Vanilla										

	Despondency	Detox	Diabetes	Diaphoretic	Diarrhea	Diet support	Diet-accompanying – inhibits cravings for sweets	Difficulty breathing	Difficulty concentrating	Difficulty falling asleep
Angelica root	X									X
Anise								X		
Arnica										
Basil										
Chamomile					X					
Cinnamon		X	X		X					
Cistus oil – lemongrass										
Dill										
Fennel										
Lavender					X					
Lemon									X	
Lemon balm										
Oregano										
Peppermint					X					
Pine needle				X						
Rose										
Rosemary						X				
St. John's wort					X					
Tea tree oil										
Thyme										
Valerian										
Vanilla							X			

	Digestion	Digestive stimulant	Diseased respiratory	Disinfectant	Dislocations	Diuretic	Dizziness	Dizziness from low blood	Dysentery	Dyspepsia	Earache and headache
Angelica root	X				X					X	
Anise						X					
Arnica						X					
Basil											
Chamomile						X					
Cinnamon	X										
Cistus oil – lemongrass						X					
Dill	X										
Fennel	X					X					
Lavender						X	X				X
Lemon	X					X					
Lemon balm							X				
Oregano	X										
Peppermint		X	X				X				
Pine needle				X		X					
Rose											
Rosemary								X			
St. John's wort									X		
Tea tree oil											
Thyme	X										
Valerian											
Vanilla											

	Earache and sore throat	Earache	Eczema	Emotional swings strong	Epilepsy	Epithelizing	Exam anxiety	Excitement	Exhaustion	Expectorant
Angelica root							X		X	X
Anise										X
Arnica										
Basil										X
Chamomile	X	X						X		
Cinnamon										
Cistus oil – lemongrass			X							
Dill										
Fennel										X
Lavender										
Lemon										
Lemon balm				X						
Oregano		X								X
Peppermint			X		X	X				
Pine needle										X
Rose										
Rosemary										
St. John's wort										
Tea tree oil										
Thyme									X	X
Valerian					X					
Vanilla										

	Expectorant	Eye discomfort	Eyesight strengthening	Fainting	Fatigue	Fear	Feet swollen	Fever	Fistulas	Fleas
Angelica root	X									
Anise							X			
Arnica										
Basil								X		
Chamomile						X		X		
Cinnamon										
Cistus oil – lemongrass										
Dill										
Fennel		X	X							
Lavender								X	X	
Lemon							X	X		
Lemon balm										
Oregano										
Peppermint				X						
Pine needle	X									
Rose					X					
Rosemary										
St. John's wort										
Tea tree oil										X
Thyme										
Valerian										
Vanilla										

	Flu	Foot perspiration	Frigidity	Frustration	Fungal diseases	Fungal diseases of the skin	Fungicidal	Fungicide	Gallstones	Gas
Angelica root	X									X
Anise										X
Arnica										
Basil										
Chamomile										X
Cinnamon								X		X
Cistus oil – lemongrass			X							
Dill										X
Fennel										X
Lavender	X									
Lemon	X								X	
Lemon balm										X
Oregano				X						
Peppermint	X							X		X
Pine needle	X									
Rose										
Rosemary										X
St. John's wort										
Tea tree oil		X					X			
Thyme										
Valerian										
Vanilla				X		X				

	Gas nervous	Gastritis	Gastrointestinal discomfort	Gastrointestinal disorders caused by stress	General hair care	Germicidal	Gingivitis	Gonorrhea	Gout
Angelica root	X	X							
Anise									
Arnica									
Basil									
Chamomile		X			X				
Cinnamon									
Cistus oil – lemongrass									
Dill									
Fennel									X
Lavender								X	
Lemon							X		X
Lemon balm			X	X					
Oregano									
Peppermint									
Pine needle									X
Rose							X		
Rosemary									
St. John's wort									X
Tea tree oil							X		
Thyme									
Valerian									
Vanilla						X			

	Granulation-enhancing	Hair greasy and dandruff	Hands swollen	Hangover	Hay fever	Head and neck pain	Head lice	Headache	Headaches and migraines	Heart disease
Angelica root										
Anise			X							
Arnica										X
Basil									X	
Chamomile								X		
Cinnamon										
Cistus oil – lemongrass										
Dill										
Fennel				X						
Lavender								X		
Lemon		X	X							
Lemon balm					X			X		
Oregano										
Peppermint	X					X		X		
Pine needle										
Rose								X		
Rosemary										
St. John's wort										
Tea tree oil							X			
Thyme										
Valerian										
Vanilla										

	Heart failure	Heart problems without organic cause	Heart trouble	Heart trouble nervous	Heavy period bleeding	Hemorrhoids	Hemostatic	Hemostatic for nosebleeds and heavy menstrual bleeding
Angelica root	X							
Anise				X				
Arnica								
Basil								
Chamomile								
Cinnamon					X		X	X
Cistus oil – lemongrass							X	
Dill								
Fennel								
Lavender				X				
Lemon							X	
Lemon balm		X	X	X				
Oregano								
Peppermint								
Pine needle								
Rose								
Rosemary								
St. John's wort						X		
Tea tree oil								
Thyme								
Valerian								
Vanilla								

	Hepatic and pancreatic insufficiency	Hepatitis	Hepatobiliary disorders	Herpes	Herpes diseases	Hiccups	Hoarseness	Hormonally balancing	Hypertension
Angelica root									
Anise									
Arnica									
Basil									
Chamomile									
Cinnamon									
Cistus oil – lemongrass									
Dill						X			
Fennel						X			
Lavender				X					X
Lemon				X			X		X
Lemon balm			X	X	X			X	X
Oregano									
Peppermint	X	X		X					
Pine needle									
Rose									
Rosemary									
St. John's wort									
Tea tree oil				X					
Thyme									
Valerian									
Vanilla									

	Hysteria	Immune and nervous deficiencies	Immune boosting	Immune stimulating	Impotence	Improvement of liver and bile activity	Indigestion
Angelica root			X				X
Anise							
Arnica							
Basil							X
Chamomile	X						X
Cinnamon			X				
Cistus oil – lemongrass				X			
Dill							
Fennel							
Lavender	X						
Lemon							
Lemon balm				X			
Oregano							
Peppermint							
Pine needle					X		
Rose							
Rosemary						X	
St. John's wort							
Tea tree oil							
Thyme		X					
Valerian							
Vanilla							

	Infected anal fistulas	Infections	Infectious diseases	Inflammation	Inflammation of the gums	Influenza infection	Inhibit tumor growth	Insect bites	Insect repellent
Angelica root			X			X			
Anise									
Arnica									
Basil								X	
Chamomile									
Cinnamon		X							
Cistus oil – lemongrass									
Dill									
Fennel									
Lavender	X	X						X	
Lemon		X				X			
Lemon balm								X	
Oregano					X		X		
Peppermint									X
Pine needle									
Rose									
Rosemary		X							
St. John's wort									
Tea tree oil		X		X				X	
Thyme									
Valerian									
Vanilla									

	Insomnia	Intelligence stimulating	Intestinal catarrh	Intestinal colic	Intestinal diseases general	Intestinal inflammation	Intestinal parasites	Irregular menstrual cycle	Irritability	Itching
Angelica root	X									
Anise				X						
Arnica										
Basil	X									
Chamomile										
Cinnamon										
Cistus oil – lemongrass										
Dill										
Fennel							X			
Lavender	X								X	
Lemon			X		X	X				X
Lemon balm	X							X		
Oregano							X			
Peppermint										X
Pine needle										
Rose										
Rosemary										
St. John's wort	X									
Tea tree oil										X
Thyme	X	X								
Valerian										
Vanilla										

	Jaundice	Kidney and biliary disorders	Kidney stimulant	Laryngitis	Leg ulcers	Leukorrhea	Libido stimulating	Lice	Lichen	Listlessness
Angelica root										
Anise										
Arnica										
Basil			X							
Chamomile	X									
Cinnamon							X			
Cistus oil – lemongrass										
Dill										
Fennel										
Lavender					X	X				
Lemon									X	
Lemon balm										
Oregano								X		
Peppermint										
Pine needle				X						
Rose										
Rosemary										X
St. John's wort		X								
Tea tree oil										
Thyme										
Valerian										
Vanilla										

	Liver and biliary disorders	Liver and spleen swelling	Liver disease	X of appetite	Lumbago	Lung	Lung ailments s	Lung diseases	Lymphatic decongestion
Angelica root									
Anise								X	
Arnica		X							
Basil				X					
Chamomile									
Cinnamon				X					
Cistus oil – lemongrass									X
Dill									
Fennel						X			
Lavender								X	
Lemon			X					X	
Lemon balm	X								
Oregano									
Peppermint					X				
Pine needle							X		
Rose									
Rosemary									
St. John's wort									
Tea tree oil									
Thyme									
Valerian									
Vanilla									

	Lymphatic drainage	Massage for tension	Massage oil for migraines and rheumatism	Melancholy	Memory enhancing	Meno-inducing	Menopause	Menostatic baths
Angelica root								
Anise								
Arnica								
Basil				X		X		
Chamomile		X						X
Cinnamon								
Cistus oil – lemongrass	X							
Dill								
Fennel						X		
Lavender								
Lemon								
Lemon balm			X				X	
Oregano								
Peppermint						X		
Pine needle								
Rose								
Rosemary					X			
St. John's wort								
Tea tree oil								
Thyme						X		
Valerian								
Vanilla								

	Menstrual cramps	Menstrual disorders – menopause	Menstrual pain (cramps)	Menstrual stimulant	Menstrual tonic slight	Mental and physical weakness	Mental exhaustion
Angelica root						X	
Anise				X			
Arnica							
Basil							X
Chamomile			X	X			
Cinnamon							
Cistus oil – lemongrass	X			X			
Dill							
Fennel							
Lavender							
Lemon							
Lemon balm	X	X					
Oregano							
Peppermint							
Pine needle							
Rose	X						
Rosemary							
St. John's wort							
Tea tree oil							
Thyme							
Valerian							
Vanilla					X		

	Mental tension	Metabolic disorders	Metabolism booster	Metabolism stimulator	Metabolism-boosting	Migraine	Mites	Moisturizing	Mood balancing
Angelica root									
Anise				X		X			
Arnica									
Basil									
Chamomile						X			
Cinnamon			X						
Cistus oil – lemongrass									
Dill									
Fennel									
Lavender						X			
Lemon		X			X	X			
Lemon balm	X					X			X
Oregano									
Peppermint									
Pine needle									
Rose						X		X	
Rosemary									
St. John's wort									
Tea tree oil							X		
Thyme									
Valerian									
Vanilla	X								

	Mood swings	Mood-enhancing	Morning sickness	Motion sickness	Mouth ulcers	Mouthwash	Mucous respiration	Multi-resistant germs	Muscle and nerve pain	Muscle cramps
Angelica root				X						X
Anise							X			
Arnica										
Basil										
Chamomile						X				
Cinnamon										
Cistus oil – lemongrass										
Dill										
Fennel										
Lavender				X						
Lemon					X					
Lemon balm			X							
Oregano								X		
Peppermint										
Pine needle										
Rose										
Rosemary	X									
St. John's wort									X	
Tea tree oil										
Thyme										
Valerian										
Vanilla		X								

	Muscle strains	Myocardial insufficiency	Nail fungus	Nausea	Nephritis	Nerve inflammation and sciatica	Nerve pain	Nerve strengthening	Nervousness
Angelica root		X		X				X	X
Anise									
Arnica									
Basil				X					X
Chamomile					X		X		X
Cinnamon			X	X					
Cistus oil – lemongrass									
Dill									
Fennel									
Lavender	X					X			
Lemon									
Lemon balm								X	X
Oregano									
Peppermint				X					
Pine needle									
Rose									
Rosemary				X					
St. John's wort								X	X
Tea tree oil			X						
Thyme							X		
Valerian								X	X
Vanilla									

	Neurasthenia	Neuritis	Neurodermatitis	Nightmares	Nocturnal awakening	Normalizes the menstrual cycle	Obesity
Angelica root							
Anise							
Arnica							
Basil							
Chamomile							
Cinnamon							
Cistus oil – lemongrass			X				
Dill							
Fennel						X	X
Lavender	X						
Lemon							X
Lemon balm				X	X		
Oregano							
Peppermint		X					
Pine needle							
Rose							
Rosemary							
St. John's wort							
Tea tree oil							
Thyme							
Valerian							
Vanilla			X				

	Over acidification of the body	Overweight	Pain relieving	Painkiller	Palpitations	Palpitations nervous	Paralysis	Parasites	Period too light or absent
Angelica root							X		
Anise									
Arnica									
Basil									X
Chamomile			X						
Cinnamon		X						X	
Cistus oil – lemongrass									
Dill									
Fennel									
Lavender			X						
Lemon	X								
Lemon balm				X		X			
Oregano			X						
Peppermint			X	X	X				
Pine needle									
Rose			X						
Rosemary									
St. John's wort				X					
Tea tree oil									
Thyme									
Valerian									
Vanilla									

	Plugged ducts	Pneumonia	Premenstrual discomfort	Prevention of colds	Prevents cancer cells from dividing	Promotes wound healing	Promoting lactation	Prostate inflammation
Angelica root								
Anise							X	
Arnica								
Basil			X					
Chamomile								
Cinnamon								
Cistus oil – lemongrass								
Dill							X	
Fennel			X				X	
Lavender								
Lemon				X				
Lemon balm	X							
Oregano		X			X			
Peppermint								X
Pine needle		X						
Rose						X		
Rosemary								
St. John's wort								
Tea tree oil								
Thyme								
Valerian								
Vanilla								

	Psoriasis	Puffiness	Purification and detoxification of the body	Purifies and drains	Purifying	Purulent wounds that heal poorly	Rapid heartbeat from low blood pressure
Angelica root							
Anise							
Arnica							
Basil							
Chamomile							
Cinnamon							
Cistus oil – lemongrass	X					X	
Dill				X			
Fennel			X		X		
Lavender	X						
Lemon		X			X		
Lemon balm							
Oregano							
Peppermint							
Pine needle							
Rose							
Rosemary							X
St. John's wort							
Tea tree oil							
Thyme							
Valerian							
Vanilla							

	Rash	Rashes	Reduces scarring	Regenerating	Regenerative	Relaxing	Relaxing with tension	Respiratory diseases	Restlessness	Restlessness inner
Angelica root										
Anise										
Arnica										
Basil										
Chamomile	X					X				
Cinnamon										
Cistus oil – lemongrass										X
Dill										
Fennel										
Lavender			X		X			X		
Lemon		X								
Lemon balm				X						
Oregano										
Peppermint										
Pine needle										
Rose							X			
Rosemary									X	
St. John's wort										
Tea tree oil										
Thyme										
Valerian										
Vanilla						X				

	Restlessness nervous	Restorative	Rheumatic complaints	Rheumatic pains	Rheumatism	Rheumatism as a rub	Rosacea	Rubella	Scabs on the scalp	Scarlet
Angelica root	X				X	X				
Anise										
Arnica										
Basil										
Chamomile					X				X	
Cinnamon					X					
Cistus oil – lemongrass								X		X
Dill										
Fennel										
Lavender			X		X		X			
Lemon					X					
Lemon balm										
Oregano										
Peppermint				X						
Pine needle		X			X					
Rose										
Rosemary										
St. John's wort					X					
Tea tree oil										
Thyme					X					
Valerian										
Vanilla										

	Scarring	Sciatica	Sciatica pain	Scurvy	Self-confidence low	Sensitivity to weather	Sexual problems	Shock	Shock states	Signs of aging
Angelica root										
Anise										
Arnica									X	
Basil										
Chamomile	X									
Cinnamon										
Cistus oil – lemongrass										
Dill										
Fennel										
Lavender										
Lemon				X	X					X
Lemon balm						X		X		
Oregano										
Peppermint			X					X		
Pine needle										
Rose										
Rosemary										
St. John's wort		X								
Tea tree oil										
Thyme										
Valerian										
Vanilla							X			

	Simple leg ulcers	Sinus infection	Sinuses blocked	Sinusitis	Skin allergies	Skin cancer	Skin care before radiotherapy	Skin conditions and blemishes
Angelica root				X				
Anise								
Arnica								
Basil								
Chamomile					X			
Cinnamon								
Cistus oil – lemongrass						X		
Dill								
Fennel								
Lavender	X							
Lemon								
Lemon balm							X	
Oregano								
Peppermint		X		X				
Pine needle		X	X					
Rose								
Rosemary								
St. John's wort								
Tea tree oil								X
Thyme								
Valerian								
Vanilla								

	Skin congested	Skin diseases	Skin diseases all	Skin flushing	Skin greasy	Skin impure	Skin inflamed	Skin inflammation	Skin itching	Skin mature
Angelica root								X		
Anise										
Arnica										
Basil										
Chamomile								X	X	
Cinnamon										
Cistus oil – lemongrass	X	X			X		X			X
Dill										
Fennel										
Lavender		X	X							
Lemon					X					
Lemon balm					X	X				
Oregano						X				
Peppermint										
Pine needle				X						
Rose										
Rosemary										
St. John's wort										
Tea tree oil										
Thyme										
Valerian										
Vanilla										

	Skin oily and impure	Skin pain	Skin problems general	Skin tired impure	Skin ulcers	Sleep disorders	Sleep-promoting	Small intestine inflammation	Soothes the scalp	Soothing
Angelica root						X				
Anise										
Arnica										
Basil										
Chamomile		X								X
Cinnamon										
Cistus oil – lemongrass										
Dill										
Fennel	X									
Lavender										
Lemon	X		X					X		
Lemon balm					X	X				X
Oregano										
Peppermint				X						
Pine needle										
Rose										
Rosemary										
St. John's wort										
Tea tree oil									X	
Thyme										
Valerian						X	X			
Vanilla										

	Sore muscles	Sore throat	Spike protein shedding	Sprains	Spring fatigue	Stabilizing	State of weakness physical	Stimulant	Stimulates blood circulation
Angelica root				X	X		X		
Anise									
Arnica									
Basil									
Chamomile									
Cinnamon									
Cistus oil – lemongrass						X			
Dill									
Fennel		X							
Lavender									
Lemon		X							
Lemon balm									
Oregano									X
Peppermint	X								
Pine needle			X					X	
Rose									X
Rosemary									
St. John's wort									
Tea tree oil		X							
Thyme									X
Valerian									
Vanilla									

	Stimulates digestion	Stimulates digestive juices	Stimulating	Stomach acidity	Stomach and intestinal diseases	Stomach and intestinal infection	Stomach and intestinal spasms
Angelica root							
Anise							
Arnica							
Basil							
Chamomile							X
Cinnamon							
Cistus oil – lemongrass							
Dill					X		
Fennel							
Lavender		X	X				
Lemon				X			
Lemon balm							
Oregano							
Peppermint							
Pine needle			X				
Rose							
Rosemary							
St. John's wort							
Tea tree oil							
Thyme						X	
Valerian							
Vanilla	X						

	Stomach and menstrual cramps	Stomach compressions	Stomach cramps	Stomach mucosa strengthening	Stomach pain	Stomach problems caused
Angelica root		X				
Anise						
Arnica						
Basil	X					X
Chamomile			X		X	
Cinnamon						
Cistus oil – lemongrass						
Dill					X	
Fennel					X	
Lavender						
Lemon						
Lemon balm			X			
Oregano				X		
Peppermint						
Pine needle						
Rose						
Rosemary						
St. John's wort						
Tea tree oil						
Thyme						
Valerian						
Vanilla						

	Stomach tonic	Stomach ulcers	Stomach upset	Stomach upset nervous	Stomach weakness	Strengthening	Strengthening	Strengthening after illness	Strengthening
Angelica root		X	X	X	X	X		X	X
Anise			X						
Arnica									
Basil	X								
Chamomile									
Cinnamon									
Cistus oil – lemongrass									
Dill									
Fennel	X								
Lavender									
Lemon		X							
Lemon balm									
Oregano									
Peppermint	X								
Pine needle						X			
Rose									
Rosemary									
St. John's wort									
Tea tree oil									
Thyme	X						X		
Valerian									
Vanilla									

	Strengthens the body's defenses against infectious diseases	Strengthens the gums as a mouthwash	Stress	Stress disorders	Stress relieving	Stretch marks	Swelling of the lymph glands
Angelica root				X			
Anise							
Arnica							
Basil			X				
Chamomile			X				
Cinnamon							
Cistus oil – lemongrass							X
Dill							
Fennel							
Lavender						X	
Lemon		X					
Lemon balm					X		
Oregano							
Peppermint							
Pine needle							
Rose							
Rosemary				X			
St. John's wort							
Tea tree oil							
Thyme	X						
Valerian							
Vanilla							

	Symptoms of stress	Teething in toddlers	Tension	Tension nervous	Thick mucus in the bronchi	Throat infections	Ticks	Tissue regenerating	Tissue tightening	Toning
Angelica root										
Anise										
Arnica										
Basil										X
Chamomile		X	X							X
Cinnamon										
Cistus oil – lemongrass	X							X		X
Dill					X					
Fennel										
Lavender										
Lemon						X				
Lemon balm	X			X					X	
Oregano										
Peppermint										
Pine needle										
Rose										
Rosemary										
St. John's wort										
Tea tree oil							X			
Thyme										
Valerian										
Vanilla										

	Tonsillitis	Toothache	Travel nausea	Trouble falling asleep	Tuberculosis	Typhoid	Ulcers	Uplifting	Urinary stones	Vaginitis
Angelica root			X							
Anise										
Arnica										
Basil										
Chamomile		X		X					X	X
Cinnamon										
Cistus oil – lemongrass										
Dill										
Fennel									X	
Lavender						X	X	X		
Lemon										
Lemon balm										
Oregano	X	X								
Peppermint		X					X			
Pine needle					X					
Rose										
Rosemary										
St. John's wort										
Tea tree oil										
Thyme					X					
Valerian										
Vanilla										

	Varicose veins	Vascular regulating	Vasoconstrictor	Vein discomfort	Venous congestion	Venous inflammation	Vermifuge	Vessel wall stabilizing	Virucide	Vomit
Angelica root										X
Anise										X
Arnica										
Basil										X
Chamomile			X							X
Cinnamon										X
Cistus oil – lemongrass								X		
Dill										X
Fennel							X			
Lavender										
Lemon	X			X	X	X				X
Lemon balm		X								
Oregano										
Peppermint									X	X
Pine needle			X							
Rose										
Rosemary										
St. John's wort										
Tea tree oil										
Thyme							X			
Valerian										
Vanilla										

	Vomit nervous	Warming	Warts	Wash or compress for badly healing wounds	Weak digestion	Weakness	Weaknesses physically and mentally
Angelica root							
Anise							
Arnica							
Basil		X		X			
Chamomile							
Cinnamon					X		
Cistus oil – lemongrass							
Dill	X	X					
Fennel							
Lavender							
Lemon			X				X
Lemon balm							
Oregano							
Peppermint							
Pine needle							
Rose							
Rosemary							
St. John's wort		X					
Tea tree oil			X				
Thyme						X	
Valerian							
Vanilla							

	Weeping rashes	Whooping cough	Worms	Wound healing	Wound healing support	Wound irrigation	Wound treatment	Wounds
Angelica root								
Anise		X						
Arnica								
Basil		X						
Chamomile		X	X	X		X		
Cinnamon								
Cistus oil – lemongrass				X				
Dill			X					
Fennel								
Lavender		X					X	X
Lemon	X							X
Lemon balm								
Oregano								
Peppermint				X				X
Pine needle								
Rose								
Rosemary				X				
St. John's wort				X				X
Tea tree oil					X			
Thyme		X						
Valerian								
Vanilla								

Oils recommendation:

I've been looking for a company for a long time that offers all the oils I recommend in good quality at a fair price. I found what I was looking for at Feeling, an Austrian company that has been around since 1991. I have linked my website below directly to it. This company delivers worldwide.

Essential oils and selected base oils are available here:

www.belly-oils.com

Classic base oils such as e.g. You can get olive oil in good health food stores or drugstores.

Production of arnica oil extract:

Ingredients: -25 g fresh arnica flowers

200ml extra virgin olive oil

Preparation: Pour the olive oil over the fresh blossoms and leave tightly closed for a month. Shake daily. Then filter the mixture and fill it into a tightly sealable container that is as dark as possible. Store in a cool place.

Index

A

G

H

L

M

References:

www.aetherische-oele.net

oelerini.com

dolce-vita.ch

www.giendl.at

de.wikipedia.org

www.karger.com

www.mimosa-massagen.de

doktorstuben.de

www.biologie-schule.de

royal-rose.de

www.xn--therisches-l-fcb7x.com

www.bio-washausen.de

satureja.de

utopia.de

gebeurtkeren.icu

www.babalawoobanifa.com

www.heilkunst-muenchen.com

www.makeup.at

www.curlychocolate.com

www.jaliya.de

life-health-balance.de

www.heilpflanzen-katalog.de

www.schule-beruf.de

www.power-soja.eu

www.wirtschaftsdeutsch.de

www.ingramcontent.com/pod-product-compliance
Lightning Source LLC
Chambersburg PA
CBHW061040250726